Alchemy of Nourishment: Unleashing the Magic of Holistic Nutrition

Holistic Nurition, Volume 1

Nancy Tran, RHN, CSS

Published by HPN, 2023.

While every precaution has been taken in the preparation of this book, the publisher assumes no responsibility for errors or omissions, or for damages resulting from the use of the information contained herein.

ALCHEMY OF NOURISHMENT: UNLEASHING THE MAGIC OF HOLISTIC NUTRITION

First edition. June 7, 2023.

Copyright © 2023 Nancy Tran, RHN, CSS.

ISBN: 979-8223215226

Written by Nancy Tran, RHN, CSS.

To my loved ones, Your unwavering support and encouragement have been the driving force behind this book. Thank you for believing in me and inspiring me to share my passion for holistic nutrition with the world. This dedication is a testament to the love and gratitude I hold in my heart for each of you. May this book serve as a token of appreciation for the countless ways you have enriched my life. Together, let us continue to embrace the journey toward vibrant health and well-being.

Biography

Nancy is a holistic nutritionist dedicated to helping individuals achieve optimal health and well-being through the power of nutrition. With a deep passion for holistic living and a strong belief in the interconnectedness of the body, mind, and spirit, Nancy has dedicated years of study and practice to holistic nutrition.

Nancy holds certifications in holistic nutrition and strength conditioning. Her expertise is creating personalized nutrition plans and food sensitivities testing that nourish the whole person, addressing physical health and emotional, mental, and spiritual well-being.

Throughout her career, Nancy has worked with clients from diverse backgrounds, helping them transform their lives through the healing power of food. Her approach goes beyond simply providing dietary guidelines but delves deeper into the root causes of health issues, considering factors such as stress, emotional well-being, and lifestyle habits.

As a holistic nutritionist, Nancy believes that food is not only fuel for the body but also medicine for the mind and nourishment for the soul. She is passionate about empowering individuals to take charge of their health, guiding them toward making sustainable dietary choices that support their unique needs and goals.

Introduction:

Welcome to "Alchemy of Nourishment: Unleashing the Magic of Holistic Nutrition" – a transformative journey towards vibrant health and well-being. In this book, I invite you to embark on a holistic nutrition adventure, where we explore food's profound impact on our bodies, minds, and overall vitality.

In today's fast-paced and stressful world, neglecting our well-being and overlooking nutrition's vital role is easy. However, I firmly believe that true wellness goes beyond counting calories or following fad diets. It involves embracing a holistic approach that nourishes our physical bodies, minds, emotions, and spirits.

Through years of experience as a holistic nutritionist, I have witnessed firsthand the remarkable transformations that occur when individuals adopt a balanced and mindful approach to their nutrition. In this book, I will guide you on a journey of self-discovery, where you will learn to harness the power of food to optimize your health, enhance your energy levels, and cultivate a profound sense of well-being.

From understanding the principles of holistic nutrition to identifying and addressing nutritional deficiencies, we will explore various often overlooked nourishment facets. We will delve into the importance of whole foods, micronutrients, and the delicate balance of macronutrients. We will also dive into the fascinating world of the gut microbiome, uncovering the secrets to digestive health and overall vitality.

But this book is about more than just the physical aspects of nutrition. It is about embracing a holistic lifestyle encompassing mindfulness, stress management, and emotional wellness. We will explore the connection between food and mental health, delve into mindful eating practices, and discuss strategies for managing emotional eating.

I am thrilled to be your guide on this holistic nutrition journey. Together, we will empower you to make informed choices, cultivate a harmonious relationship with food, and unlock your body's innate ability to heal and thrive. So, get ready to nourish your body, energize your mind, and embark toward radiant well-being.

Let's begin this transformative adventure toward optimal nutrition and vibrant health!

With warmth and enthusiasm,

Nancy Tran

"Alchemy of Nourishment: Unleashing the Magic of Holistic Nutrition"

It combines mystery, transformation, and holistic nutrition as a transformative process. Here's an analysis of the title:

Alchemy of Nourishment: "Alchemy" carries a sense of transformation, turning something ordinary into something extraordinary. It suggests that nourishment goes beyond mere sustenance and can profoundly affect the body and mind.

Unleashing the Magic: "Unleashing the magic" creates a sense of wonder and excitement. It implies that something is enchanting and extraordinary about the power of holistic nutrition and its potential to bring about positive changes.

Holistic Nutrition: This term emphasizes the comprehensive and integrated approach to nutrition, addressing not only the physical aspects but also the mental, emotional, and spiritual well-being.

The Essence of Holistic Nutrition

5

What is Holistic Nutrition?

Holistic nutrition is a method of nourishing the body that considers the interdependence of various aspects of health and well-being, such as physical, mental, emotional, and spiritual factors. It recognizes that optimal nutrition entails more than just focusing on the nutrients in food and emphasizes the significance of a balanced lifestyle and overall wellness.

Fundamental principles of holistic nutrition include:

Bio-individuality: They recognize that people have different dietary demands based on age, genetics, lifestyle, and health concerns. There is no such thing as a one-size-fits-all approach to nutrition.

Whole Foods: Consuming nutrient-dense, unprocessed, and minimally refined foods. Whole foods are high in essential nutrients, phytochemicals, and antioxidants, all promoting general health.

Nutrient Balance: Balancing macronutrients (carbohydrates, proteins, and fats) with micronutrients (vitamins and minerals) to meet individual demands and promote optimal biological processes.

Mind-Body Connection: understanding the impact of ideas, emotions, stress, and lifestyle on general health and healthy digestion and absorption. Maintaining optimal nutrition requires addressing mental and emotional well-being.

Digestive Health: Recognizing the importance of a healthy digestive system for nutrient absorption and overall well-being. Supporting gut health through a balanced diet, probiotics, and fibre is a fundamental aspect of holistic nutrition.

Individualized Approach: Tailoring nutrition recommendations to each person's unique needs, goals, and preferences. This includes considering food sensitivities, allergies, personal beliefs and cultural influences related to food.

Holistic Lifestyle: Promoting a balanced lifestyle that includes regular physical activity, stress management techniques, quality sleep, and mindful eating practices to enhance overall well-being.

Holistic nutrition empowers individuals to actively participate in their health and make informed choices supporting their well-being. It encourages a holistic view of nutrition that encompasses not only the physical aspects of food but also the mental, emotional, and spiritual aspects of nourishment.

Nourishing Your Body and Mind

CHAPTER 1: THE POWER OF BALANCED NUTRITION

The Importance of a Balanced Diet

A balanced diet is crucial for maintaining good health and preventing chronic diseases. This is because it provides the body with nutrients, energy, and fibre to support optimal bodily functions. Here are some of the reasons why a balanced diet is essential:

Nutrient Adequacy: A balanced diet provides the body with all the essential nutrients required for optimal functioning, including carbohydrates, proteins, fats, vitamins, and minerals. These nutrients support various bodily functions, such as energy production, cell repair, immune function, and brain health.

Disease Prevention: A balanced diet rich in whole foods, including fruits, vegetables, whole grains, lean proteins, and healthy fats, can help prevent chronic diseases such as heart disease, diabetes, and some cancers. These foods are rich in antioxidants, phytochemicals, and other compounds supporting cellular health and preventing harmful free radicals damage.

Weight Management: Eating a balanced diet can help maintain a healthy weight, reducing the risk of obesity and related conditions such as heart disease, diabetes, and high blood pressure. A balanced diet can also help regulate hunger and satiety hormones, reducing the risk of overeating and cravings.

Gut Health: A balanced diet with fibre-rich foods, probiotics, and fermented foods supports gut health and the microbiome. A healthy gut microbiome is essential for proper nutrient absorption, immune function, and overall health.

Mental Health: A balanced diet with foods rich in omega-3 fatty acids, B vitamins, and antioxidants can support mental health and reduce the risk of depression, anxiety, and other mood disorders.

Energy and Vitality: A balanced diet gives the body the power to support physical activity, mental alertness, and overall vitality. Eating a balanced diet can help reduce fatigue and improve overall quality of life.

Longevity: A balanced diet rich in whole foods and low in processed foods is associated with a longer lifespan and reduced risk of chronic diseases.

In summary, a balanced diet is essential for optimal health and well-being. It provides the body with the necessary nutrients for optimal functioning, disease prevention, weight management, gut health, mental health, energy, and longevity. Therefore, individuals can achieve and maintain optimal health and wellness by prioritizing a balanced diet.

Assessing Your Current Health and Nutritional Status

Assessing your current health and nutritional status is essential in understanding your needs and determining areas that may require improvement. Here are some key aspects to consider when evaluating your health and nutritional status:

Medical History: Review your medical history, including past or present health conditions, allergies, surgeries, medications, and treatments. This information provides valuable insight into your overall health and may influence your nutritional needs.

Physical Examinations: Consider any recent physical examinations or check-ups you've had. These may include measurements such as height, weight, body mass index (BMI), blood pressure, and blood work results. These measurements can help assess your general health and identify potential nutritional deficiencies or imbalances.

Dietary Assessment: Evaluate your current dietary habits and patterns. Keep a food diary for a few days to track everything you eat and drink, including portion sizes and preparation methods. This assessment helps identify any nutrient gaps, excessive intake of certain nutrients, and areas where dietary improvements can be made.

Nutrient Intake: Analyze your nutrient intake using your food diary. Compare it to recommended daily allowances or dietary guidelines for essential nutrients such as vitamins, minerals, carbohydrates, proteins, fats, and fibre. This assessment can highlight any deficiencies or imbalances that need to be addressed.

Symptoms and Energy Levels: Consider any specific symptoms or health concerns you may be experiencing, such as fatigue, digestive issues, skin problems, or mood disturbances. These symptoms can provide clues about potential nutritional deficiencies or intolerances.

Emotional and Mental Well-being: Assess your emotional and mental well-being, as they can significantly impact your nutritional status. Stress, anxiety, depression, and eating disorders can affect your appetite, food choices, and nutrient absorption. Identifying any emotional or mental health challenges can guide you toward appropriate support and strategies.

Lifestyle Factors: Consider your lifestyle factors, including physical activity, sleep patterns, stress levels, and smoking or alcohol consumption. These factors can influence your nutritional needs and overall health status.

Professional Guidance: Consult with a healthcare professional, such as a registered dietitian or a holistic nutritionist. They can conduct a comprehensive assessment, provide personalized recommendations, and help you interpret your health and nutritional status more accurately.

By assessing your current health and nutritional status, you gain insights into areas that require attention and develop a foundation for creating a personalized nutrition plan. Remember that the assessment process should be ongoing, as health and nutritional needs can change over time. Regular evaluations allow you to adjust and ensure you're meeting your evolving health goals.

Identifying Nutritional Deficiencies

Identifying nutritional deficiencies is vital in assessing your overall health and well-being. Here are some common signs and symptoms that may indicate potential nutrient deficiencies:

Fatigue and Weakness: A lack of energy and persistent fatigue can indicate deficiencies in various nutrients, including iron, magnesium, vitamin B12, and vitamin D.

Poor Wound Healing: Slow wound healing or frequent infections may indicate deficiencies in vitamin C, vitamin A, zinc, and protein.

Brittle Hair and Nails: Weak, brittle hair and nails can indicate nutrient deficiencies like biotin, vitamin E, zinc, and iron.

Skin Issues: Dry skin, acne, eczema, or other skin problems may be associated with deficiencies in essential fatty acids, vitamin A, vitamin E, vitamin C, or zinc.

Pale Complexion: A pale or washed-out complexion may indicate iron deficiency, leading to anemia.

Poor Concentration and Cognitive Function: Difficulty focusing, poor memory, and cognitive impairment can be related to nutrient deficiencies such as omega-3 fatty acids, B vitamins, magnesium, and zinc.

Bone Health Issues: Frequent fractures, osteoporosis, or tooth decay can indicate deficiencies in calcium, vitamin D, vitamin K, and magnesium.

Muscle Cramps: Frequent muscle cramps and spasms may be associated with deficiencies in electrolytes (such as potassium, magnesium, and calcium) or vitamin D.

Digestive Problems: Issues like bloating, constipation, or diarrhea can be related to deficiencies in fibre, probiotics, or digestive enzymes.

Changes in Appetite: Loss of appetite or persistent food cravings may indicate deficiencies in specific nutrients, such as zinc, magnesium, vitamin C, or vitamin B12.

It's important to note that these symptoms can have multiple causes, and professional evaluation is crucial to identify nutritional deficiencies accurately. If you suspect nutrient deficiencies, consult a healthcare professional or registered dietitian/ Nutritionists who can conduct appropriate tests, analyze your dietary intake, and provide personalized recommendations to address any deficiencies detected.

A comprehensive assessment, including a thorough review of medical history, physical examinations, and laboratory tests, is often necessary to determine specific nutrient deficiencies accurately.

Chapter 2: Unlocking the Magic of Holistic Nutrition

The Mind-Body Connection

The mind-body connection refers to the intricate relationship and interaction between our mental and emotional state (mind) and physical health and well-being (body). It recognizes that our thoughts, emotions, beliefs, and attitudes can influence our physical health; conversely, our physical health can impact our mental and emotional state.

Here are key aspects and examples of the mind-body connection:

Stress and Physical Health: Psychological stress can manifest as physical symptoms or exacerbate existing health conditions. For instance, chronic stress can contribute to high blood pressure, weakened immune function, digestive disorders, headaches, and sleep disturbances.

Placebo Effect: The placebo effect demonstrates the power of the mind in influencing physical responses. When individuals believe they are receiving a beneficial treatment, even a placebo (an inactive substance), they may experience tangible improvements in symptoms. This highlights the impact of the mind's beliefs and expectations on the body's response.

Psychosomatic Illnesses: Certain physical conditions are influenced by or have a significant psychological component. Examples include tension headaches, irritable bowel syndrome (IBS), fibromyalgia, and some skin disorders. In addition, emotional distress and psychological factors can contribute to these conditions' development, severity, or exacerbation.

Mindfulness and Pain Management: Mindfulness practices, such as meditation and deep breathing, have been shown to reduce pain perception and improve pain management. Individuals can positively influence their physical experience of pain by cultivating present-moment awareness and non-judgmental acceptance.

Emotional Well-being and Immune Function: Research suggests positive emotions, such as happiness, optimism, and a sense of purpose, can boost immune function and overall health. On the other hand, chronic negative emotions, such as anger, anxiety, and depression, can weaken immune responses and increase vulnerability to illness.

Mind-Body Practices: Various mind-body practices, such as yoga, tai chi, and qigong, emphasize integrating physical movements, breath control, and mental focus. These practices promote relaxation, stress reduction, flexibility, balance, and well-being.

Cognitive-behavioural Therapy (CBT): CBT is a therapeutic approach that recognizes the connection between thoughts, emotions, and behaviours. By addressing and modifying negative or maladaptive thought patterns, CBT can positively impact mental health conditions and improve physical symptoms related to stress and illness.

Recognizing and nurturing the mind-body connection is crucial for holistic health and well-being. It highlights the importance of promoting positive mental and emotional states, managing stress effectively, and integrating practices supporting psychological and physical health. By acknowledging the mind-body connection, individuals can take a proactive approach to optimize their overall well-being.

Detoxification and Cleansing

Detoxification and cleansing are terms commonly used in health and wellness to describe practices or interventions to eliminate toxins or promote the body's natural detoxification processes. While these terms are often used interchangeably, it's essential to understand their meanings and the evidence behind them.

Detoxification refers to the body's natural process of eliminating or neutralizing toxins. The liver, kidneys, digestive system, skin, and lungs are the primary organs involved in detoxification. They work together to filter and eliminate waste products, metabolic byproducts, environmental toxins, and harmful substances.

Cleansing typically refers to specific practices or interventions to support or enhance the body's detoxification processes. These practices can include various dietary approaches, fasting, juicing, herbal supplements, colon cleansing, or other methods to eliminate toxins from the body.

It's important to note that the body has sophisticated mechanisms to detoxify and eliminate toxins naturally. The liver plays a central role in detoxification by metabolizing and removing toxins, while the kidneys filter waste products from the blood and excrete them in urine. The digestive system also plays a crucial role in eliminating waste and toxins through bowel movements.

While some detoxification practices may have short-term benefits or make individuals feel better, it's essential to approach them with caution and consider the following:

Scientific Evidence: The evidence supporting the efficacy and safety of many detoxification and cleansing practices is often limited or inconclusive. Some approaches may need more scientific validation or rely on anecdotal evidence.

Individual Variations: Each person's detoxification capacity and needs are unique. Age, health status, genetics, lifestyle, and exposure to toxins can influence the body's detoxification ability. Therefore, what may work for one person may not be suitable or effective for another.

Nutritional Considerations: Some detoxification approaches may involve restrictive diets or fasting, potentially leading to nutrient deficiencies or imbalances if not carefully planned. It's vital to ensure that any detoxification practice includes an adequate intake of essential nutrients.

Potential Risks: Certain detoxification practices, such as extreme fasting, prolonged juice cleanses, or aggressive colon cleansing, can carry risks and may be harmful, especially for individuals with specific health conditions or on certain medications. Therefore, consulting a healthcare professional before undertaking any intensive detoxification program is advisable.

Instead of relying on drastic detoxification or cleansing interventions, focusing on long-term lifestyle habits that support the body's natural detoxification processes is generally recommended. These habits include:

- Consuming a balanced, whole-foods-based diet that provides essential nutrients and antioxidants.

- Staying well-hydrated to support kidney function and promote the elimination of waste products.

- Engaging in regular physical activity to support circulation, sweating, and lymphatic flow.

- Minimizing exposure to environmental toxins and pollutants when possible.

- Managing stress levels and incorporating stress-reduction techniques, as chronic stress can impact the body's detoxification processes.

- Prioritizing healthy sleep patterns, as sleep is vital in supporting overall health and detoxification.

Remember, it's always best to consult with a healthcare professional or registered dietitian/ nutritionist before embarking on any detoxification or cleansing program to ensure it is safe and appropriate for your needs.

Balancing pH Levels

Balancing pH levels refers to maintaining the proper acid-alkaline balance in the body. The pH scale measures the acidity or alkalinity of a substance and ranges from 0 to 14, with 7 being considered neutral. A pH below 7 is acidic, while an above 7 is alkaline.

Different systems and organs have specific pH levels crucial for optimal functioning in the human body. For example, the blood pH is tightly regulated within a narrow range of 7.35 to 7.45, slightly alkaline. Deviations from this range can have adverse effects on health.

Here are some tips to help balance pH levels in the body:

Consume a Balanced Diet: A diet rich in whole, unprocessed foods can help maintain proper pH balance. Focus on fruits, vegetables, whole grains, lean proteins, and healthy fats. These foods tend to have an alkaline effect on the body.

Increase Alkaline Foods: Incorporate more alkaline-forming foods, such as leafy green vegetables, cruciferous vegetables (broccoli, cauliflower), citrus fruits, berries, and nuts. These foods can help counteract acidity in the body.

Reduce Acidic Foods: Limit or avoid highly acidic foods, such as processed foods, refined sugars, excessive amounts of animal proteins, refined grains, and carbonated beverages. These foods can contribute to an acidic environment in the body.

Stay Hydrated: Drinking plenty of water helps maintain proper hydration and supports the body's natural detoxification processes. Aim for adequate daily water intake to support overall health.

Moderate Alcohol and Caffeine: Excessive alcohol consumption and high caffeine intake can increase acidity in the body. Moderate your consumption of these beverages to maintain a balanced pH.

Manage Stress: Chronic stress can contribute to acidity in the body. Practice stress management techniques such as meditation, deep breathing exercises, yoga, or engaging in activities you enjoy to promote relaxation and balance.

Exercise Regularly: Regular physical activity helps maintain overall health and can contribute to pH balance. Choose activities that you enjoy and engage in them consistently.

It's important to note that while dietary choices can impact pH levels in the body, the body has robust mechanisms to regulate pH within the appropriate ranges. Therefore, the focus should be on overall healthy eating habits rather than obsessing over individual pH levels of foods.

Suppose you have specific concerns about pH levels or suspect an imbalance. In that case, it's advisable to consult with a healthcare professional or registered dietitian /nutritionist who can provide personalized guidance based on your individual needs and health status.

CHAPTER 3: THE FOUNDATION OF OPTIMAL HEALTH: WHOLE FOODS

Understanding Whole Foods

Understanding whole foods is essential for making informed and healthy dietary choices. Whole foods are minimally processed or unprocessed foods that are as close to their natural state as possible. They are typically nutrient-dense and provide many essential vitamins, minerals, fibre, and phytochemicals. Here are vital aspects to consider when understanding whole foods:

Definition: Whole foods refer to foods that have undergone minimal processing or refining, preserving their natural nutrient content. They are typically found naturally or require minimal preparation before consumption.

Nutrient Density: Whole foods are rich in essential nutrients, including vitamins, minerals, antioxidants, and fibre. They offer various health-promoting benefits, support optimal body function, and help prevent nutrient deficiencies.

Examples of Whole Foods: Whole foods include fruits, vegetables, whole grains, legumes, nuts, seeds, lean meats, fish, poultry, and dairy products that are minimally processed or unprocessed. Examples include apples, spinach, quinoa, lentils, almonds, wild-caught salmon, and natural yogurt.

Fibre Content: Whole foods are excellent sources of dietary fibre, which aids in digestion, promotes satiety and helps regulate blood sugar levels. Fibre also supports a healthy gut microbiome and can contribute to heart health.

Phytochemicals and Antioxidants: Whole foods are abundant in phytochemicals, natural compounds found in plants with numerous health benefits. These phytochemicals, including antioxidants, can protect against chronic diseases, reduce inflammation, and support overall well-being.

Minimally Processed vs. Highly Processed Foods: Minimally processed whole foods retain their natural structure and nutrient composition. On the other hand, highly processed foods undergo extensive refining, often resulting in removing essential nutrients and adding additives, preservatives, and artificial ingredients.

Benefits of Whole Foods: Incorporating whole foods into your diet offers several advantages. They provide essential nutrients in their natural form, support overall health, contribute to a balanced diet, and can help prevent chronic diseases like heart disease, diabetes, and certain types of cancer.

Meal Planning with Whole Foods: Prioritizing whole foods in meal planning involves incorporating a variety of fruits, vegetables, whole grains, lean proteins, and healthy fats into your meals. Aim to consume various plant-based foods and minimize reliance on highly processed or refined foods.

Remember that while whole foods form the foundation of a healthy diet, individual nutritional needs may vary. Consulting with a registered dietitian/nutritionist can provide personalized guidance and help you create a well-balanced meal plan based on your dietary requirements and health goals.

Nutrient-Dense Foods for Optimal Health

Incorporating nutrient-dense foods into your diet is crucial for optimal health as they provide a wide array of essential nutrients while minimizing empty calories. Here are some nutrient-dense foods to consider:

Leafy Green Vegetables: Leafy greens like spinach, kale, Swiss chard, and collard greens are packed with vitamins A, C, K, and folate, as well as minerals like iron and calcium. They are also rich in fibre and antioxidants.

Cruciferous Vegetables: Vegetables such as broccoli, cauliflower, Brussels sprouts, and cabbage are excellent sources of vitamins C, K, and folate. They also contain phytochemicals that have been associated with potential cancer-fighting properties.

Berries: Berries like blueberries, strawberries, raspberries, and blackberries are low in calories. Full of antioxidants, fibre, and vitamins. They are particularly rich in vitamin C and various phytochemicals.

Fish: Fatty fish such as salmon, mackerel, sardines, and trout are excellent sources of omega-3 fatty acids, which are beneficial for heart health and brain function. They also provide high-quality protein and essential nutrients like vitamin D and selenium.

Legumes: Legumes, including lentils, chickpeas, black beans, and kidney beans, are rich in protein, fibre, vitamins, and minerals. They are also a good source of plant-based iron and are beneficial for promoting satiety and maintaining stable blood sugar levels.

Nuts and Seeds: Almonds, walnuts, chia seeds, flaxseeds, and hemp seeds are packed with healthy fats, fibre, vitamins and minerals. They are also a good source of plant-based protein and can contribute to heart health.

Whole Grains: Whole grains like quinoa, brown rice, oats, and whole wheat provide fibre, B vitamins, minerals, and antioxidants. They are less processed than refined grains and can help regulate blood sugar levels and support digestive health.

Greek Yogurt: Greek yogurt is a good source of protein, calcium, probiotics, and vitamin B12. Opt for plain Greek yogurt without added sugars and customize it with fresh fruits and nuts for added flavour and nutrients.

Colourful Vegetables and Fruits: Incorporate a variety of colourful vegetables and fruits into your diet as they provide different vitamins, minerals, antioxidants, and phytochemicals. Examples include carrots, bell peppers, sweet potatoes, oranges, and papayas.

Lean Protein: Choose lean sources of protein such as poultry, eggs, tofu, tempeh, and lean cuts of meat. These provide essential amino acids for muscle repair and growth.

Remember, a balanced and varied diet with a wide range of nutrient-dense foods is critical to optimal nutrition. When planning meals, it's also essential to consider individual dietary needs and specific health conditions or allergies. Consulting with a registered dietitian/ nutritionist can provide personalized guidance to help you create a well-rounded and nutrient-rich eating plan tailored to your needs.

Incorporating Superfoods into Your Diet

Incorporating superfoods into your diet is a great way to boost your nutrient intake and support your overall health. Superfoods are nutrient-dense foods rich in vitamins, minerals, antioxidants, and other beneficial compounds. Here are some superfoods you can consider incorporating into your diet:

Berries: Berries, such as blueberries, strawberries, raspberries, and blackberries, are packed with antioxidants, fibre, and vitamins. As a result, they have been linked to various health benefits, including improved cognitive function and reduced inflammation.

Leafy Green Vegetables: Leafy greens like spinach, kale, Swiss chard, and collard greens are rich in vitamins A, C, and K, as well as minerals like iron and calcium. They are also a good source of fibre and antioxidants.

Avocado: Avocado is a nutrient-dense fruit that is rich in heart-healthy monounsaturated fats, fibre, potassium, and vitamins K, C, E, and B vitamins. It can be enjoyed in salads, smoothies, or as a spread on toast.

Chia Seeds: Chia seeds are a great source of omega-3 fatty acids, fibre, protein, and antioxidants. They can be added to smoothies, oatmeal, yogurt, or an egg substitute in baking.

Quinoa: Quinoa is a gluten-free whole grain packed with protein, fibre, and essential amino acids. It is also rich in minerals like magnesium, iron, and zinc. Quinoa can be used as a base for salads, served as a side dish, or incorporated into soups and stews.

Greek Yogurt: Greek yogurt is a good source of protein, calcium, probiotics, and vitamin B12. Opt for plain Greek yogurt without added sugars and customize it with fresh fruits and nuts for added flavour and nutrients.

Turmeric: Turmeric is a spice known for its anti-inflammatory properties. It contains a compound called curcumin, which has been studied for potential health benefits. Turmeric can be used in curries, stir-fries, smoothies, or as a tea.

Salmon: Salmon is fatty fish rich in omega-3 fatty acids, which are beneficial for heart health and brain function. It is also a good source of high-quality protein and contains vitamins D and B12.

Nuts and Seeds: Almonds, walnuts, chia seeds, flaxseeds, and hemp seeds are nutrient-dense and packed with healthy fats, fibre, vitamins, minerals, and antioxidants. They make great snacks or can be added to smoothies, salads, or homemade granola.

Green Tea: Green tea is rich in antioxidants, particularly catechins, associated with various health benefits, including improved brain function and a reduced risk of chronic diseases.

Remember, while incorporating superfoods into your diet can provide nutritional benefits, focusing on overall dietary balance and variety is essential. No single food can provide all the nutrients your body needs. So instead, aim for a well-rounded diet with diverse nutrient-dense foods to support optimal health.

CHAPTER 4: EMBRACING ORGANIC AND LOCALLY SOURCED FOODS

The Benefits of Organic and Locally Sourced Foods

Organic and locally sourced foods offer several benefits for your health and the environment. Here are some key advantages of choosing organic and locally sourced foods:

Benefits of Organic Foods:

Reduced Exposure to Pesticides: Organic farming practices avoid using synthetic pesticides, herbicides, and fertilizers. Choosing organic foods reduces your exposure to potentially harmful chemicals and pesticide residues.

Nutrient Content: Organic farming methods focus on soil health and natural fertilizers, which can result in higher nutrient content in organic produce. Some studies suggest that certain organic foods may have higher levels of vitamins, minerals, and antioxidants.

No GMOs: Organic foods are produced without genetically modified organisms (GMOs). If avoiding GMOs is your priority, choosing organic products ensures you consume foods free from genetically engineered ingredients.

Environmental Impact: Organic farming practices promote sustainability and prioritize soil health, biodiversity, and water conservation. By supporting organic farming, you contribute to the protection of ecosystems and the reduction of pollution.

Animal Welfare: Organic animal products, such as organic meat, eggs, and dairy, come from animals raised in more humane conditions. Organic standards require that animals have access to outdoor space, exercise, and a diet free from antibiotics and growth hormones.

Benefits of Locally Sourced Foods:

Freshness and Flavor: Locally sourced foods are often harvested at peak ripeness and transported shorter distances. This results in fresher produce with better flavour and nutritional quality.

Support Local Economy: Buying locally sourced foods supports local farmers and producers, contributing to the local economy's vitality. In addition, it helps sustain small-scale agriculture, preserves farmland, and fosters community connections.

Environmental Impact: By choosing locally sourced foods, you reduce the carbon footprint associated with long-distance transportation. Buying from local farmers reduces the need for fuel consumption, packaging materials, and refrigeration.

Seasonal Eating: Locally sourced foods encourage seasonal eating, where you consume foods that are naturally available during specific times of the year. This promotes diversity in your diet and supports a more sustainable food system.

Transparency and Relationships: Buying locally lets you connect directly with farmers and producers. You can learn about their farming practices, ask questions about food production, and develop a deeper understanding of where your food comes from.

It's important to note that while organic and locally sourced foods offer advantages, they may not always be accessible or affordable for everyone. Making the best choices for your health and the environment involves balancing considerations based on individual circumstances.

Making Informed Food Choices

Our modern world is bombarded with an overwhelming array of food choices. With clever marketing tactics and conflicting information, navigating the sea of options and making choices that truly support our health and well-being can be challenging. However, by arming ourselves with knowledge and adopting a mindful approach, we can make informed food choices that nourish our bodies and promote optimal vitality. In this chapter, we will explore the key factors to consider when making food choices and provide practical strategies to help you navigate the complex food landscape.

Understanding Food Labels:

Decoding Nutrition Labels: Learn how to read and interpret nutrition labels to make informed decisions about the nutritional content of packaged foods.

Unveiling Ingredient Lists: Understand the importance of ingredient lists and how to identify additives, preservatives, and other potentially harmful substances.

Identifying Hidden Sugars and Artificial Sweeteners: Discover the various names of added sugars and artificial sweeteners, and learn how to spot them on food labels.

Grasping Food Quality:

Organic vs. Conventional: Explore the differences between organic and conventionally grown foods and the potential benefits of choosing organic options.

Locally Sourced and Seasonal Foods: Discover the advantages of choosing locally sourced and seasonal foods, including freshness, reduced environmental impact, and support for local communities.

GMOs and Food Safety: Gain insights into genetically modified organisms (GMOs) and considerations for food safety.

Diving into Dietary Patterns:

Whole Foods Approach: Embrace the power of whole foods and the benefits of incorporating minimally processed, nutrient-dense options into your diet.

Plant-Based Diets: Explore the advantages of plant-based diets and learn how to incorporate more plant-based meals into your eating habits.

Mindful Meat Consumption: Understand the importance of conscious meat choices, including selecting high-quality, ethically sourced, and sustainably raised options.

Considering Individual Needs and Preferences:

Personalized Nutrition: Recognize that nutrition is not a one-size-fits-all approach and learn how to tailor your food choices to your unique needs and preferences.

Allergies, Sensitivities, and Intolerances: Discover strategies for navigating food allergies, sensitivities, and intolerances, including reading labels, identifying common allergens, and finding suitable alternatives.

Cultural and Ethical Considerations: Explore the impact of cultural and ethical factors on food choices and gain insights into aligning your dietary practices with your values.

By making informed food choices, you have the power to nourish your body and mind, promote overall well-being, and support a sustainable and healthy future. Remember, every bite you take is an opportunity to feed yourself and positively impact your health. With the knowledge and strategies in this chapter, you can approach food choices with confidence, mindfulness, and the intention of nurturing your body and mind.

Part II: Macro- and Micronutrients for Well-Being

CHAPTER 5: UNVEILING THE POWER OF MACRONUTRIENTS

Carbohydrates: Fueling Your Body

Carbohydrates are a vital energy source for our bodies, serving as the primary fuel for various physiological functions. However, not all carbohydrates are created equal, and understanding their different forms and effects on the body is essential for making informed dietary choices. In this chapter, we will explore carbohydrates, their role in providing energy, the different types of carbohydrates, and strategies for incorporating them into a balanced and nourishing diet.

The Role of Carbohydrates in the Body:

Energy Source: Understand how carbohydrates are converted into glucose, which the body uses as fuel to support physical and cognitive functions.

Glycogen Storage: Learn about glycogen, the storage form of glucose in the body, and its role in maintaining stable blood sugar levels.

Carbohydrates and Exercise: Discover how carbohydrates impact athletic performance and exercise recovery, and explore strategies for fueling your workouts effectively.

Simple and Complex Carbohydrates:

Simple Carbohydrates: Explore the characteristics of simple carbohydrates, such as sugars and refined grains, and their quick absorption by the body.

Complex Carbohydrates: Learn about complex carbohydrates found in whole grains, legumes, and starchy vegetables, which provide sustained energy and essential nutrients.

The Fiber Factor:

Soluble vs. Insoluble Fiber: Understand the different types of dietary fibre and their effects on digestion, satiety, and overall health.

Benefits of Fiber: Explore the numerous benefits of fibre, including improved digestion, cholesterol management, and blood sugar regulation.

Increasing Fiber Intake: Discover practical ways to incorporate fibre-rich foods into your diet, such as whole grains, fruits, vegetables, and legumes.

Balancing Carbohydrate Intake:

Understanding Glycemic Index and Load: Learn about carbohydrates' glycemic index and glycemic load and how they affect blood sugar levels and overall health.

Carbohydrates and Weight Management: Explore strategies for maintaining a healthy weight through mindful carbohydrate choices, portion control, and balanced meals.

Individual Needs and Carbohydrate Intake: Consider factors such as activity level, health conditions, and personal goals when determining the appropriate amount and types of carbohydrates for your body.

Healthy Carbohydrate Sources:

Whole Grains: Discover a variety of nutrient-dense whole grains, such as quinoa, brown rice, and oats, and their health benefits.

Fruits and Vegetables: Explore different fruits and vegetables' carbohydrate content and nutritional value, and learn how to incorporate them into a well-rounded diet.

Legumes and Beans: Learn about legumes and beans' carbohydrate and fibre content, which provide a sustainable energy source and essential nutrients.

Carbohydrates are vital in fueling our bodies and supporting optimal health and performance. By understanding the different types of carbohydrates, their effects on blood sugar, and the importance of fibre, you can make informed choices to nourish your body with suitable sources and amounts of carbohydrates. Remember, a balanced and mindful approach to carbohydrate intake can provide sustained energy, support overall well-being, and contribute to a healthy and vibrant life.

Proteins: Building Blocks for Health

Proteins are the building blocks of life, playing a crucial role in various physiological processes within our bodies. From supporting growth and repair to maintaining a robust immune system, proteins are essential for overall health and vitality. This chapter will explore the importance of proteins, their functions, sources, and strategies for incorporating them into a balanced and nourishing diet.

The Importance of Proteins:

Structural Support: Understand how proteins contribute to the formation and maintenance of tissues, including muscles, bones, and skin.

Enzymes and Metabolic Processes: Explore the role of proteins as enzymes, facilitating biochemical reactions and metabolic processes within the body.

Immune System Function: Learn how proteins help to strengthen the immune system and support a healthy defence against pathogens.

Essential Amino Acids:

Understanding Amino Acids: Discover the fundamental units of proteins, amino acids, and the distinction between essential and non-essential amino acids.

Complete and Incomplete Proteins: Learn about complete protein sources that contain all essential amino acids and incomplete protein sources that lack one or more essential amino acids.

Complementary Protein Pairing: Explore combining incomplete protein sources to form a complete amino acid profile and maximize protein quality.

Protein Sources for Optimal Nutrition:

Animal-Based Proteins: Discover high-quality protein sources from animal products, such as lean meats, poultry, fish, eggs, and dairy, and their nutrient profiles.

Plant-Based Proteins: Explore a variety of plant-based protein sources, including legumes, nuts, seeds, whole grains, and soy products, and their unique nutritional benefits.

Balancing Protein Intake: Learn about the recommended daily protein intake and strategies for balancing protein sources to meet your nutritional needs.

Protein for Special Dietary Considerations:

Vegetarian and Vegan Protein Sources: Gain insights into meeting protein needs on a vegetarian or vegan diet, including plant-based protein-rich foods and supplementation options.

Protein and Weight Management: Understand the role of protein in supporting weight loss, satiety, and muscle maintenance, and explore strategies for incorporating protein into a balanced weight management plan.

Protein and Aging: Explore the importance of protein for older adults to support muscle mass, strength, and overall health.

Cooking and Preparation Tips:

Cooking Methods for Protein Retention: Discover cooking techniques that preserve proteins' nutritional value and quality.

Flavorful and Healthy Protein Choices: Learn about healthy seasoning options and creative ways to add flavour to protein-rich dishes without relying on unhealthy additives.

Meal Planning with Protein: Explore ideas for incorporating protein-rich foods into balanced meals and snacks throughout the day.

Proteins are the backbone of our body's structure and function, vital in supporting growth, repair, and overall health. By incorporating various protein sources into your diet, you can ensure you provide your body with the essential amino acids it needs for optimal nutrition. Whether you choose animal-based or plant-based proteins, remember that balance and variety are crucial. Embrace the power of proteins and make them a cornerstone of your well-rounded, nourishing diet.

Fats: Essential for Vitality

Fats often get a bad reputation, but they are essential for our overall health and vitality. From providing energy to supporting cell function and nutrient absorption, fats are crucial in numerous physiological processes within our bodies. In this chapter, we will explore the importance of fats, the different types of fats, their functions, and strategies for incorporating them into a balanced and nourishing diet.

Understanding Dietary Fats:

Types of Dietary Fats: Explore the different types of fats, including saturated, unsaturated (monounsaturated and polyunsaturated), and trans fats, and their effects on health.

Differentiating Between "Good" and "Bad" Fats: Learn how to identify healthy fats that support optimal health and well-being while minimizing the consumption of unhealthy fats.

Functions and Benefits of Fats:

Energy and Nutrient Storage: Understand how fats serve as a concentrated energy source and aid in storing fat-soluble vitamins.

Cell Structure and Function: Explore how fats are integral to cell membranes' structure and function, helping maintain their integrity and facilitate cellular processes.

Hormone Regulation: Learn about the role of fats in hormone production, balance, and overall endocrine health.

Essential Fatty Acids:

Omega-3 Fatty Acids: Discover the importance of omega-3 fatty acids for brain health, cardiovascular function, and reducing inflammation.

Omega-6 Fatty Acids: Understand the role of omega-6 fatty acids and the importance of achieving a proper balance with omega-3 fatty acids.

Sources of Essential Fatty Acids: Explore food rich in omega-3 and omega-6 fatty acids, such as fatty fish, nuts, seeds, and plant-based oils.

Incorporating Healthy Fats into Your Diet:

Cooking Oils: Learn about different cooking oils and their smoke points to make informed choices for other cooking methods.

Nuts and Seeds: Discover the nutritional benefits of nuts and seeds, such as almonds, walnuts, chia seeds, and flaxseeds, and how to incorporate them into your diet.

Avocado and Coconut: Explore the unique properties of avocado and coconut, which offer healthy fats and additional health benefits.

Balancing Fat Intake:

Portion Control and Moderation: Understand the importance of portion control when consuming fats, as they are calorically dense.

Healthy Fat Substitutes: Discover alternatives to unhealthy fats, such as replacing butter with avocado or using Greek yogurt instead of mayonnaise in recipes.

Individual Needs and Fat Intake: Consider factors such as age, activity level, and specific health conditions when determining the appropriate amount and types of fats for your body.

Fats are essential to a balanced and nourishing diet, supporting energy production, cell function, and overall health. By understanding the different types of fats and their operations and incorporating healthy sources into your meals, you can harness the power of fats to optimize your vitality and well-being. Embrace the role of fats in your diet and enjoy the benefits they provide to fuel your body and support optimal health.

CHAPTER 6: MICRONUTRIENTS: VITAMINS AND MINERALS

Understanding Micronutrients

Micronutrients, including vitamins and minerals, are essential for our bodies to function optimally. While they are required in smaller quantities than macronutrients, their role in supporting various physiological processes is equally vital. This chapter will delve into the worries, exploring the different types, their functions, food sources, and the importance of maintaining a balanced intake for overall health and well-being.

The Role of Micronutrients:

Vitamins: Learn about the diverse functions of vitamins, including their involvement in metabolism, immune function, bone health, and antioxidant activity.

Minerals: Understand the importance of minerals in processes such as muscle function, nerve transmission, hormone regulation, and maintaining fluid balance.

Water-Soluble Vitamins:

Vitamin C: Explore the benefits of vitamin C in supporting immune function, collagen synthesis, antioxidant activity, and iron absorption. Discover food sources rich in vitamin C.

B Vitamins: Dive into B vitamins, including thiamin, riboflavin, niacin, vitamin B6, folate, vitamin B12, biotin, and pantothenic acid. Learn about their functions, food sources, and potential health benefits.

Fat-Soluble Vitamins:

Vitamin A: Understand the role of vitamin A in vision, immune function, and cell growth. Discover food sources rich in preformed vitamin A and beta-carotene.

Vitamin D: Learn about the importance of vitamin D for bone health, immune function, and its sources, including sunlight exposure and dietary sources.

Vitamin E: Explore the antioxidant properties of vitamin E and its role in protecting cells from oxidative damage. Discover food sources abundant in vitamin E.

Vitamin K: Understand the significance of vitamin K in blood clotting and bone health. Learn about food sources rich in vitamin K1 and vitamin K2.

Essential Minerals:

Calcium: Discover the importance of calcium in building and maintaining strong bones and teeth and its role in muscle function and nerve transmission. Learn about dietary sources of calcium.

Iron: Explore the role of iron in oxygen transport, energy production, and its association with preventing iron-deficiency anemia. Identify iron-rich food sources.

Zinc: Understand the functions of zinc in immune function, growth and development, and wound healing. Discover food sources abundant in zinc.

Magnesium: Learn about the role of magnesium in muscle function, nerve transmission, energy metabolism, and food sources.

Selenium: Explore the antioxidant properties of selenium and its role in thyroid function and immune health. Discover dietary sources of selenium.

Achieving Micronutrient Balance:

Whole Foods Approach: Embrace a diet rich in whole, unprocessed foods to naturally obtain a wide array of micronutrients.

Supplementation: Understand when supplementation may be necessary and how to make informed choices.

Factors Affecting Micronutrient Absorption: Explore factors that impact the absorption and utilization of micronutrients, such as food preparation, gut health, and interactions with other nutrients.

Micronutrients are the unsung heroes that support numerous biochemical reactions and contribute to our overall health and well-being. By understanding the different types of fats and their functions and incorporating healthy sources into your meals, you can harness the power of fats to optimize your vitality and well-being. So embrace the role of fats in your diet and enjoy their benefits to fuel your body and support optimal health.

Essential Vitamins for Optimal Health

Vitamins are organic compounds that are vital for our overall health and well-being. They are crucial in various physiological processes, including energy production, immune function, and cellular growth and repair. In this chapter, we will explore the importance of essential vitamins for optimal health, their processes, food sources, and strategies for ensuring an adequate intake.

Vitamin A:

Functions and Benefits: Understand the role of vitamin A in vision, immune function, and cell growth and differentiation.

Food Sources: Explore natural sources of vitamin A, including carrots, sweet potatoes, leafy green vegetables, and liver.

Vitamin B Complex:

Types and Functions: Discover the different types of B vitamins (B1, B2, B3, B5, B6, B7, B9, B12) and their specific functions in energy production, nervous system health, and red blood cell formation.

Food Sources: Learn about foods rich in B vitamins, such as whole grains, legumes, leafy green vegetables, eggs, and meat.

Vitamin C:

Functions and Benefits: Explore the antioxidant properties of vitamin C, its role in collagen synthesis, and its impact on immune health.

Food Sources: Discover vitamin C-rich foods, including citrus fruits, berries, bell peppers, and broccoli.

Vitamin D:

Functions and Benefits: Understand the role of vitamin D in bone health, immune function, and calcium absorption.

Sources of Vitamin D: Learn about natural sources of vitamin D, including sunlight exposure and dietary sources such as fatty fish, fortified dairy products, and mushrooms.

Vitamin E:

Functions and Benefits: Explore the antioxidant properties of vitamin E, its role in protecting cell membranes, and its potential benefits for heart health.

Food Sources: Discover vitamin E-rich foods, including nuts, seeds, vegetable oils, and leafy green vegetables.

Vitamin K:

Functions and Benefits: Understand the role of vitamin K in blood clotting, bone health, and potential anti-inflammatory effects.

Food Sources: Learn about food sources of vitamin K, such as leafy green vegetables, broccoli, Brussels sprouts, and fermented foods.

Essential vitamins are vital for maintaining optimal health and well-being. By understanding the functions and food sources of essential vitamins like A, B complex, C, D, E, and K, you can ensure your body receives the necessary nutrients for its various processes. Embrace the power of these vitamins and make informed food choices to support your overall health and vitality.

Minerals: The Foundations of Wellness

Minerals are essential nutrients for maintaining overall wellness and supporting various bodily functions. For example, they are involved in bone health, nerve transmission, muscle function, and enzyme activity. In this chapter, we will explore the importance of minerals for optimal health, their processes, food sources, and strategies for ensuring an adequate intake.

Macro Minerals:

Calcium: Discover the significance of calcium for strong bones and teeth, muscle function, and nerve transmission. Learn about calcium-rich food sources like dairy products, leafy green vegetables, and fortified plant-based alternatives.

Magnesium: Understand the role of magnesium in energy production, muscle relaxation, and bone health. Explore food sources of magnesium, including nuts, seeds, whole grains, and leafy green vegetables.

Potassium: Learn about potassium's role in maintaining fluid balance, nerve function, and blood pressure regulation. Discover potassium-rich foods like bananas, avocados, citrus fruits, and legumes.

Trace Minerals:

Iron: Explore the importance of iron in oxygen transport, energy production, and immune function. Learn about iron-rich food sources like lean meats, legumes, dark leafy greens, and fortified cereals.

Zinc: Understand the role of zinc in immune function, wound healing, and DNA synthesis. Discover zinc-rich foods such as oysters, red meat, poultry, nuts, and seeds.

Selenium: Discover the antioxidant properties of selenium and its role in thyroid function and immune support. Explore selenium-rich foods like Brazil nuts, seafood, whole grains, and eggs.

Electrolytes:

Sodium: Learn about the role of sodium in fluid balance, nerve function, and muscle contraction. Understand the importance of moderating sodium intake and choosing healthier sources.

Potassium: Revisit the role of potassium as an electrolyte and its importance for maintaining fluid balance and supporting proper muscle and nerve function.

Other Electrolytes: Explore other electrolytes, such as chloride and phosphate, and their significance for maintaining proper bodily functions.

Absorption and Bioavailability:

Factors Affecting Mineral Absorption: Understand how diet, digestive health, and interactions with other nutrients can impact mineral absorption.

Enhancing Mineral Absorption: Learn about strategies to enhance mineral absorption, such as consuming vitamin C-rich foods with iron-rich foods and pairing calcium sources with vitamin D.

Minerals are the foundations of wellness, playing crucial roles in various bodily functions. By understanding the importance of macro minerals like calcium, magnesium, and potassium, trace minerals like iron, zinc, and selenium, and electrolytes like sodium and potassium, you can make informed food choices to support optimal health. Embrace the power of minerals and nourish your body with nutrient-rich foods to lay a strong foundation for overall wellness.

CHAPTER 7: THE FIBER CONNECTION

The Importance of Fiber

Fibre is an essential component of a healthy diet, yet it is often overlooked. It is crucial in maintaining digestive health, regulating blood sugar levels, supporting weight management, and reducing the risk of chronic diseases. In this chapter, we will explore the importance of fibre, its different types, recommended intake, health benefits, and strategies for incorporating fibre-rich foods into your diet.

Understanding Fiber:

Soluble vs. Insoluble Fiber: Learn about the two main fibre types, their characteristics, and how they interact with the body.

Dietary Fiber vs. Functional Fiber: Understand the difference between dietary fibre, which occurs naturally in foods, and functional fibre, added to foods for health benefits.

Health Benefits of Fiber:

Digestive Health: Discover how fibre promotes regular bowel movements, prevents constipation, and supports a healthy gut microbiome.

Blood Sugar Regulation: Learn how fibre slows down glucose absorption, helps maintain stable blood sugar levels, and reduces the risk of diabetes.

Weight Management: Explore how fibre provides a feeling of fullness, aids in appetite control, and supports healthy weight management.

Heart Health: Understand how fibre helps lower cholesterol levels, reduces the risk of heart disease, and promotes overall cardiovascular health.

Food Sources of Fiber:

Whole Grains: Discover fibre-rich whole grains such as oats, quinoa, brown rice, and whole wheat.

Fruits and Vegetables: Learn about fibre-packed fruits and vegetables like berries, apples, broccoli, and leafy greens.

Legumes and Pulses: Explore the fibre content of legumes such as lentils, chickpeas, black beans, and kidney beans.

Nuts and Seeds: Understand how nuts and seeds like almonds, chia seeds, flaxseeds, and pumpkin seeds can contribute to your daily fibre intake.

Tips for Increasing Fiber Intake:

Gradual Increase: Learn how to increase fibre intake to avoid digestive discomfort gradually.

Reading Food Labels: Understand how to read food labels to identify high-fibre foods and make informed choices.

Meal Planning and Preparation: Discover strategies for incorporating fibre-rich foods into your meal planning and preparation routines.

Fibre is a vital nutrient that offers numerous health benefits. By understanding its importance, different types, and food sources, you can make informed choices to increase your fibre intake and support your overall health and well-being. So embrace the power of fibre and enjoy a diet rich in fibre-packed foods to optimize your digestive health, regulate blood sugar levels, manage weight, and reduce the risk of chronic diseases.

High-Fiber Foods for Digestive Health

A diet rich in fibre is essential for maintaining optimal digestive health. Fibre promotes regular bowel movements, supports a healthy gut microbiome, aids in weight management, and reduces the risk of chronic diseases. In this chapter, we will explore a variety of high-fibre foods that can help you improve your digestive health and enjoy the benefits of a fibre-rich diet.

Whole Grains:

Oats: Discover oats' fibre content and health benefits, and explore different ways to incorporate them into your meals and snacks.

Quinoa: Learn about quinoa as a high-fibre alternative to traditional grains and explore creative ways to incorporate it into your diet.

Brown Rice: Understand the fibre content of brown rice and how it compares to white rice. Discover delicious recipes that feature brown rice.

Fruits and Vegetables:

Berries: Explore the fibre-rich properties of raspberries, blackberries, and blueberries, and learn how to enjoy them in various dishes.

Apples: Discover the benefits of apples' soluble and insoluble fibre, and learn creative ways to include them in your diet.

Cruciferous Vegetables: Learn about fibre-packed cruciferous vegetables like broccoli, cauliflower, and Brussels sprouts, and discover tasty recipes featuring these nutritious veggies.

Legumes and Pulses:

Lentils: Understand the fibre content of lentils and explore delicious lentil-based recipes that can boost your fibre intake.

Chickpeas: Discover the fibre benefits of chickpeas and learn how to incorporate them into salads, soups, and homemade hummus.

Black Beans: Learn about the high fibre content of black beans and explore recipes that highlight this nutritious legume.

Nuts and Seeds:

Almonds: Discover almonds' fibre content and other health benefits, and learn how to incorporate them into your snacks and meals.

Chia Seeds: Explore chia seeds' fibre and omega-3 fatty acid content and learn how to use them in puddings, smoothies, and baked goods.

Flaxseeds: Understand the fibre and omega-3 benefits of flaxseeds and discover ways to incorporate them into your diet for added nutrition.

Incorporating high-fibre foods into your diet is essential for promoting digestive health and overall well-being. You can increase your fibre intake by including whole grains, fruits and vegetables, legumes and pulses, nuts and seeds and enjoy the numerous health benefits of a fibre-rich diet. Embrace these high-fibre foods and create delicious, nourishing meals that support your digestive health and contribute to your overall wellness.

Foods that Support Digestive Health

Maintaining a healthy digestive system is crucial for overall well-being and optimal nutrient absorption. The food we eat plays a significant role in supporting digestive health. In this chapter, we will explore a variety of foods that promote a healthy digestive system and relieve common digestive issues.

Fiber-Rich Foods:

Whole Grains: Discover the benefits of whole grains such as oats, quinoa, and brown rice, which are fibre-rich and promote regular bowel movements.

Fruits and Vegetables: Learn about the fibre content of fruits and vegetables and how they contribute to a healthy gut and digestive function.

Legumes: Explore the digestive benefits of legumes like lentils, chickpeas, and black beans, which provide both fibre and plant-based protein.

Fermented Foods:

Yogurt and Kefir: Understand how these probiotic-rich dairy products can improve digestion and support a healthy gut microbiome.

Sauerkraut and Kimchi: Discover the benefits of fermented vegetables, which provide beneficial bacteria and enzymes for digestive health.

Ginger and Peppermint:

Ginger: Learn about ginger's anti-inflammatory and soothing properties that can alleviate digestive discomfort and promote healthy digestion.

Peppermint: Explore how peppermint can help relax the gastrointestinal tract muscles, easing symptoms such as bloating and indigestion.

Papaya and Pineapple:

Papaya: Discover the enzyme papain found in papaya, which aids in protein digestion and helps prevent digestive issues.

Pineapple: Learn about bromelain, an enzyme found in pineapple that assists in breaking down proteins and reducing inflammation in the gut.

Bone Broth:

Nutrient-Rich Broth: Understand the benefits of bone broth, which contains collagen, amino acids, and minerals that support gut healing and repair.

Herbal Teas:

Peppermint Tea: Explore the soothing properties of peppermint tea for digestive discomfort and relaxation of the gastrointestinal tract.

Chamomile Tea: Learn about the calming effects of chamomile tea on the digestive system, reducing inflammation and promoting relaxation.

Incorporating digestive-friendly foods into your diet can significantly enhance your digestive health, alleviate common digestive issues, and support a balanced gut microbiome. By including fibre-rich foods, fermented foods, ginger, peppermint, papaya, pineapple, bone broth, and herbal teas in your meals and snacks, you can promote optimal digestion and overall well-being. So, experiment with these foods, discover the ones that work best for your digestive system and enjoy the benefits of a healthy gut.

Part III: Nurturing Your Digestive System

CHAPTER 8: THE ROLE OF THE DIGESTIVE SYSTEM

Understanding Digestion and Absorption

Digestion and absorption are fundamental processes that allow our bodies to break down food and extract essential nutrients for energy, growth, and overall health. Understanding how these processes work is critical to optimizing our nutritional intake and supporting a healthy digestive system. This chapter will delve into the intricate mechanisms of digestion and absorption, exploring the organs involved, the role of enzymes, and the journey of nutrients through our bodies.

The Digestive System:

Overview of Digestive Organs: Explore the various organs involved in the digestive process, including the mouth, esophagus, stomach, small intestine, and large intestine.

The Role of Enzymes: Understand how digestive enzymes facilitate the breakdown of carbohydrates, proteins, and fats into smaller components for absorption.

Carbohydrate Digestion and Absorption:

Salivary Amylase: Learn about the initial digestion of carbohydrates in the mouth by salivary amylase.

Pancreatic Amylase: Discover how pancreatic amylase further breaks down carbohydrates in the small intestine.

Absorption of Glucose: Understand how glucose is absorbed into the bloodstream and utilized by the body for energy.

Protein Digestion and Absorption:

Stomach Acid and Pepsin: Explore how the stomach's hydrochloric acid and the enzyme pepsin initiate protein digestion.

Pancreatic Enzymes: Learn how pancreatic enzymes, such as trypsin and chymotrypsin, break down proteins into amino acids.

Absorption of Amino Acids: Understand the process of amino acid absorption in the small intestine and its utilization throughout the body.

Fat Digestion and Absorption:

Bile and Emulsification: Discover how bile aids in the small intestine's emulsification and breakdown of fats.

Pancreatic Lipase: Learn about the role of pancreatic lipase in breaking down fats into fatty acids and glycerol.

Micelle Formation and Absorption: Understand how micelles facilitate the absorption of fatty acids and glycerol into the intestinal cells.

Vitamins and Minerals:

Absorption of Water-Soluble Vitamins: Explore how water-soluble vitamins are absorbed in the small intestine and their transportation throughout the body.

Absorption of Fat-Soluble Vitamins: Learn about the unique process of absorbing fat-soluble vitamins with the help of dietary fat.

Mineral Absorption: Understand the different mechanisms involved in the absorption of minerals, including passive diffusion and active transport.

Digestion and absorption are intricate processes that allow our bodies to extract and utilize essential nutrients for optimal health. By understanding how our digestive system works, the role of enzymes, and the absorption of carbohydrates, proteins, fats, vitamins, and minerals, we can make informed choices to support our digestive health and ensure proper nutrient intake. Embrace this knowledge and nourish your body by optimizing digestion and absorption for overall well-being.

Supporting Gut Health

A healthy gut is essential for overall well-being. It plays a significant role in digestion, nutrient absorption, immune function, and mental health. Therefore, supporting your gut health can profoundly impact your overall wellness. This chapter will explore various strategies and practices that can help you nurture and support a thriving gut microbiome.

The Gut Microbiome:

Understanding the Microbiome: Learn about the trillions of microorganisms in your gut and their essential functions.

Gut-Brain Axis: Explore the connection between the gut and the brain and how the microbiome influences mental health and well-being.

Diet and Gut Health:

Fiber-Rich Foods: Discover how incorporating fibre-rich foods promotes a diverse and healthy gut microbiome.

Fermented Foods: Learn about the benefits of fermented foods like yogurt, sauerkraut, and kimchi for gut health.

Prebiotic Foods: Understand the role of prebiotics in nourishing beneficial gut bacteria and promoting a balanced microbiome.

Probiotics and Gut Health:

Probiotic Supplements: Explore the use of probiotic supplements to introduce beneficial bacteria into your gut.

Probiotic-Rich Foods: Discover natural sources of probiotics such as kefir, kombucha, and miso and how they can enhance gut health.

Lifestyle Factors for Gut Health:

Stress Management: Understand the impact of stress on gut health and explore stress reduction techniques to support a healthy microbiome.

Physical Activity: Learn how regular exercise contributes to gut health and promotes a diverse microbiome.

Sleep and Gut Health: Explore the connection between sleep quality and gut health, and discover tips for improving your sleep hygiene.

Avoiding Gut Disruptors:

Antibiotic Use: Understand the effects of antibiotics on the gut microbiome and explore strategies to minimize their impact.

Processed Foods and Artificial Additives: Learn about the potentially harmful effects of processed foods and artificial additives on gut health.

Nurturing your gut health is a vital aspect of maintaining overall wellness. By adopting a gut-friendly diet, incorporating probiotics, managing stress, engaging in regular physical activity, and avoiding gut disruptors, you can support a thriving gut microbiome, and experience improved digestion, enhanced nutrient absorption, strengthened immunity, and even better mental health. Embrace these practices and prioritize your gut health to optimize your overall well-being.

CHAPTER 9: CULTIVATING A HEALTHY GUT MICROBIOME

The Gut-Brain Connection

The connection between our gut and brain goes beyond the digestive system. It is a complex and fascinating relationship crucial to our overall well-being. In this chapter, we will delve into the intricacies of the gut-brain connection and explore how the health of our gut can impact our mental and emotional well-being.

Anatomy of the Gut-Brain Connection:

The Vagus Nerve: Understand the vagus nerve's role in transmitting signals between the gut and brain.

Enteric Nervous System: Explore the enteric nervous system, often called the "second brain," and its influence on gut function and communication with the central nervous system.

Gut Health and Mental Health:

Serotonin Production: Discover how most serotonin, a neurotransmitter associated with mood regulation, is produced in the gut.

Inflammation and Mood Disorders: Understand the impact of gut inflammation on mental health conditions such as anxiety and depression.

Gut Microbiome and Mental Health:

Microbiota Composition: Learn about the diverse community of microorganisms in the gut and their influence on brain function and behaviour.

Gut Microbes and Neurotransmitters: Explore the connection between gut microbes and the production of neurotransmitters, such as GABA and dopamine.

Stress and the Gut-Brain Axis:

Stress and Gut Function: Understand how stress affects gut motility, permeability, and microbial balance.

Mind-Body Techniques: Discover mindfulness, meditation, and other stress management techniques that positively impact the gut-brain axis.

Strategies for a Healthy Gut-Brain Connection:

Gut-Friendly Diet: Learn about dietary choices that support a healthy gut microbiome and promote optimal brain function.

Probiotics and Psychobiotics: Explore the potential benefits of probiotics and psychobiotics in improving mental health through gut modulation.

Lifestyle Factors: Discover additional lifestyle factors, such as regular exercise, adequate sleep, and social connection, that contribute to a balanced gut-brain link.

The gut-brain connection is a fascinating and intricate relationship that highlights the interdependence of our digestive system and mental well-being. By understanding the influence of gut health on mental health, we can adopt strategies to nurture and support this vital connection. For example, we can optimize our overall well-being, improve mood regulation, and enhance cognitive function through a gut-friendly diet, stress management techniques, and lifestyle choices that promote a healthy gut microbiome.

Healing Leaky Gut Syndrome

Leaky gut syndrome, also known as increased intestinal permeability, is characterized by the weakening of the intestinal lining, leading to the leakage of toxins, undigested food particles, and bacteria into the bloodstream. This can trigger various health issues and inflammation throughout the body. This chapter will explore the causes, symptoms, and strategies for healing leaky gut syndrome and restoring gut integrity for better overall health.

Understanding Leaky Gut Syndrome:

Intestinal Permeability: Learn about the role of the intestinal lining in maintaining a barrier between the gut and the bloodstream.

Causes and Contributing Factors: Explore the factors that can contribute to the leaky gut syndrome, including diet, stress, medications, and certain medical conditions.

Recognizing the Symptoms:

Digestive Symptoms: Understand how leaky gut syndrome can manifest as bloating, gas, diarrhea, constipation, and abdominal pain.

Systemic Symptoms: Discover the potential systemic symptoms such as fatigue, brain fog, joint pain, skin rashes, and autoimmune conditions.

Dietary Approaches for Healing:

Elimination Diet: Learn how an elimination diet can help identify trigger foods that exacerbate leaky gut syndrome and promote gut healing.

Gut-Healing Foods: Explore foods such as bone broth, fermented vegetables, collagen-rich foods, and omega-3 fatty acids supporting gut repair.

Anti-Inflammatory Diet: Understand the importance of reducing inflammation by including anti-inflammatory foods like turmeric, ginger, and leafy greens.

Gut-Healing Supplements:

Probiotics: Explore the role of probiotics in restoring a healthy balance of gut bacteria and improving gut integrity.

L-Glutamine: Learn about the benefits of L-glutamine, an amino acid that supports intestinal cell regeneration and healing.

Digestive Enzymes: Discover how digestive enzymes can assist in the breakdown of food and alleviate stress on the gut lining.

Lifestyle Factors for Healing:

Stress Reduction: Explore stress management techniques such as meditation, deep breathing exercises, and regular exercise to support gut healing.

Sleep and Rest: Understand the importance of quality sleep and adequate rest in promoting gut repair and overall well-being.

Exercise and Movement: Learn how regular physical activity can enhance digestion, reduce inflammation, and support gut health.

Healing leaky gut syndrome requires a comprehensive approach that addresses the underlying causes, supports gut healing, and promotes overall wellness. Adopting a gut-healing diet, incorporating specific supplements, managing stress, prioritizing sleep, and engaging in regular physical activity can restore gut integrity, alleviate symptoms, and improve overall health and well-being. Embrace these strategies and empower yourself to heal your gut and thrive.

CHAPTER 10: ACHIEVING BLOOD SUGAR BALANCE

Blood Sugar Regulation and Health

Balancing blood sugar levels is essential for maintaining optimal health and well-being. Conversely, fluctuations in blood sugar can lead to various health issues, including diabetes, obesity, fatigue, and hormonal imbalances. In this chapter, we will explore the importance of blood sugar regulation, understand the impact of imbalanced blood sugar levels on overall health, and discover strategies to promote stable energy and well-being.

Understanding Blood Sugar:

The Role of Glucose: Learn about glucose, the body's primary energy source, and its role in blood sugar regulation.

Insulin and Glucagon: Explore the functions of insulin and glucagon, the hormones responsible for regulating blood sugar levels.

The Consequences of Imbalanced Blood Sugar:

Diabetes and Insulin Resistance: Understand the link between imbalanced blood sugar and the development of type 2 diabetes and insulin resistance.

Energy Imbalances: Discover how unstable blood sugar levels can lead to energy highs and crashes, affecting mood, focus, and productivity.

Weight Management: Explore the connection between blood sugar imbalances and weight gain or difficulty in losing weight.

Strategies for Balancing Blood Sugar:

Balanced Meals: Learn the importance of including a combination of complex carbohydrates, proteins, and healthy fats in each meal for stable blood sugar levels.

Portion Control: Understand the significance of portion control in managing blood sugar levels and preventing overeating.

Glycemic Index: Discover how the glycemic index of foods can help guide food choices and manage blood sugar levels.

Fiber-Rich Foods: Explore the role of fibre in slowing down glucose absorption and promoting stable blood sugar levels.

Regular Physical Activity: Learn how exercise can improve insulin sensitivity and promote better blood sugar control.

Mindful Eating for Blood Sugar Regulation:

Awareness and Mindful Choices: Understand the importance of mindful eating, paying attention to hunger cues, and making conscious food choices.

Emotional Eating: Explore strategies to manage emotional eating and prevent blood sugar spikes caused by stress or emotional triggers.

Blood Sugar-Supportive Nutrients:

Chromium and Magnesium: Discover the role of these essential minerals in blood sugar regulation and insulin sensitivity.

Cinnamon and Fenugreek: Learn about the potential benefits of these herbs and spices in improving blood sugar control.

Omega-3 Fatty Acids: Explore how omega-3 fatty acids can support insulin sensitivity and reduce inflammation.

Maintaining stable blood sugar levels is crucial for overall health and well-being. By understanding the impact of imbalanced blood sugar on the body and implementing strategies for blood sugar regulation, such as balanced meals, portion control, regular physical activity, mindful eating, and incorporating blood sugar-supportive nutrients, you can promote stable energy levels, prevent chronic diseases, and optimize your overall health. Embrace these strategies and take charge of your blood sugar for a healthier and more vibrant life.

Nutritional Strategies for Balanced Blood Sugar Levels

Maintaining balanced blood sugar levels is essential for overall health and well-being. However, when blood sugar levels are consistently elevated or erratic, it can lead to various health issues, including insulin resistance, diabetes, weight gain, and energy imbalances. This chapter will explore effective nutritional strategies to promote balanced blood sugar levels and support overall health.

Emphasize Complex Carbohydrates:

Whole Grains: Learn about the benefits of whole grains such as brown rice, quinoa, and oats, which provide complex carbohydrates and fibre for the slow and steady release of glucose into the bloodstream.

Legumes: Discover the importance of incorporating legumes like lentils, chickpeas, and beans, which are high in fibre and protein, into your meals for sustained energy and stable blood sugar levels.

Include High-Fiber Foods:

Fruits and Vegetables: Explore the fibre content of a variety of fruits and vegetables, such as berries, leafy greens, and cruciferous vegetables, which can help slow down the absorption of glucose and promote stable blood sugar levels.

Chia Seeds and Flaxseeds: Learn about these seeds' fibre and omega-3 fatty acid content, which can support blood sugar regulation when added to meals and snacks.

———

Opt for Healthy Fats:

Avocados: Discover the benefits of avocados, rich in monounsaturated fats and fibre, for improved blood sugar control and satiety.

Nuts and Seeds: Understand how incorporating nuts and seeds, such as almonds, walnuts, and chia seeds, can provide healthy fats, protein, and fibre to help balance blood sugar levels.

Balance Meals with Protein:

Lean Poultry and Fish: Learn about the importance of including lean protein sources, such as chicken, turkey, and fish, in your meals to promote stable blood sugar levels and feelings of fullness.

Plant-Based Proteins: Explore options like tofu, tempeh, and legumes, which provide plant-based protein and fibre for sustained energy and blood sugar control.

Control Portion Sizes:

Mindful Eating: Understand the significance of mindful eating, pay attention to hunger and fullness cues, and practice portion control to avoid overeating and blood sugar spikes.

Balanced Plate Method: Discover a practical approach to building balanced meals by dividing your plate into portions of complex carbohydrates, lean proteins, and vegetables.

Avoid or Limit Sugary and Processed Foods:

Sugary Beverages and Desserts: Understand the impact of high-sugar foods and beverages on blood sugar levels and the importance of minimizing consumption.

Processed Foods: Learn about the potential adverse effects of processed foods, often high in refined carbohydrates and added sugars, on blood sugar regulation.

Incorporating these nutritional strategies into your daily routine supports balanced blood sugar levels, improves insulin sensitivity, and promotes overall health and well-being. Emphasizing complex carbohydrates, high-fibre foods, healthy fats, and lean proteins while controlling portion sizes and minimizing sugary and processed foods will help you maintain stable energy levels, prevent blood sugar imbalances, and support your long-term health goals. Empower yourself with these nutritional strategies and enjoy the benefits of balanced blood sugar levels.

Part IV: Holistic Nutrition for Mental and Emotional Well-Being

CHAPTER 11: NOURISHMENT FOR STRESS MANAGEMENT

The Impact of Stress on Health

In today's fast-paced and demanding world, stress has become a standard part of our lives. Unfortunately, while some pressure is daily and motivating, chronic and unmanaged stress can harm our health and well-being. In this chapter, we will explore the profound effects of stress on our physical and mental health and discuss strategies to manage and reduce stress for optimal well-being effectively.

Understanding Stress:

The Stress Response: Learn about the body's physiological and hormonal response to stress, including releasing cortisol and adrenaline.

Acute vs. Chronic Stress: Differentiate between acute stress, which is short-term and manageable, and chronic stress, which persists over a prolonged period and can lead to adverse health consequences.

The Physical Effects of Chronic Stress:

Cardiovascular Health: Explore the link between chronic stress and increased risk of hypertension, heart disease, and other cardiovascular conditions.

Immune System: Understand how chronic stress can weaken the immune system, making individuals more susceptible to infections and illnesses.

Digestive Health: Discover how stress can disrupt digestion, leading to symptoms such as indigestion, stomach ulcers, and irritable bowel syndrome (IBS).

Hormonal Imbalances: Learn about the impact of chronic stress on hormonal regulation, including disruptions in the adrenal glands, thyroid function, and reproductive hormones.

Mental and Emotional Effects of Chronic Stress:

Anxiety and Depression: Understand the connection between chronic stress and developing anxiety disorders and depression.

Cognitive Function: Explore how chronic stress can impair memory, concentration, and decision-making abilities.

Sleep Disturbances: Learn about the relationship between stress and sleep problems, including insomnia and sleep disturbances.

Effective Stress Management Strategies:

Relaxation Techniques: Discover relaxation techniques such as deep breathing exercises, meditation, and progressive muscle relaxation to reduce stress levels.

Physical Activity: Understand the benefits of regular exercise in managing and reducing stress, including releasing endorphins and promoting overall well-being.

Healthy Lifestyle Habits: Explore the importance of maintaining a balanced diet, getting sufficient sleep, and practicing self-care activities to manage stress.

Time Management and Prioritization: Learn practical strategies for organizing and managing time to reduce stress and increase productivity.

Seeking Support: Understand the importance of seeking social support from friends, family, or professional counsellors to cope with chronic stress effectively.

Chronic stress can significantly impact our physical, mental, and emotional well-being. By understanding the effects of stress on our health and implementing effective stress management strategies, we can minimize its negative impact and cultivate a healthier and more balanced life. Prioritizing relaxation techniques, engaging in regular physical activity, adopting healthy lifestyle habits, managing time effectively, and seeking support will empower us to cope with stress and promote overall well-being. Take control of pressure and embrace a healthier and more resilient life.

Nutritional Support for Stress Management

In our modern, fast-paced lives, stress has become an everyday companion. While eliminating stress is impossible, we can support our bodies and minds through proper nutrition. This chapter will explore the powerful connection between nutrition and stress management. Discover how certain foods and nutrients can help reduce stress, promote relaxation, and support overall well-being.

The Stress-Reducing Role of Macronutrients:

Complex Carbohydrates: Learn how complex carbohydrates, such as whole grains, legumes, and vegetables, can increase serotonin production and promote a calming effect on the body.

High-Quality Proteins: Explore the importance of consuming lean proteins, including poultry, fish, tofu, and legumes, to support the production of neurotransmitters and stabilize blood sugar levels for improved mood and energy.

Healthy Fats: Understand the role of healthy fats from sources like avocados, nuts, seeds, and fatty fish in reducing inflammation, supporting brain health, and providing a sense of satiety.

Essential Micronutrients for Stress Management:

B Vitamins: Discover how B vitamins, particularly B6, B12, and folate, are vital in neurotransmitter synthesis and stress hormone regulation.

Magnesium: Learn about the calming effects of magnesium on the nervous system and its role in reducing anxiety and promoting relaxation.

Vitamin C: Explore the antioxidant properties of vitamin C and its role in supporting the adrenal glands and reducing the negative impact of stress on the body.

Omega-3 Fatty Acids: Understand the benefits of omega-3 fatty acids for reducing inflammation, supporting brain health, and improving mood.

Adaptogenic Herbs and Foods:

Ashwagandha: Discover the stress-reducing properties of ashwagandha, an adaptogenic herb that helps the body adapt to stress and promotes relaxation.

Turmeric: Learn about turmeric's anti-inflammatory and mood-balancing effects, which can support stress management and overall well-being.

Green Tea: Explore green tea's calming and antioxidant properties, which contain the amino acid L-theanine, known for its relaxing mental effects.

Gut-Brain Axis and Probiotics:

Gut-Brain Connection: Understand the intricate relationship between the gut and the brain and how maintaining a healthy gut microbiome through probiotics can positively impact stress levels and mental health.

Probiotic-Rich Foods: Explore fermented foods such as yogurt, kefir, sauerkraut, and kimchi, which provide beneficial bacteria to support gut health and improve stress response.

Mindful Eating for Stress Reduction:

Mindful Eating Practices: Learn techniques for practicing mindful eating, such as slowing down, savouring each bite, and paying attention to hunger and fullness cues, to reduce stress and promote a healthy relationship with food.

Emotional Eating Awareness: Understand the connection between stress and emotional eating and explore strategies for developing healthier coping mechanisms.

Incorporating these nutritional strategies into your daily routine can support your body's resilience against stress, enhance relaxation, and improve overall well-being. Emphasizing the right balance of macronutrients, incorporating essential micronutrients, incorporating adaptogenic herbs and foods, nurturing the gut-brain axis, and practicing mindful eating can profoundly impact stress management. Remember, nourishing your body with the right foods is a powerful tool for supporting your mind during times of stress. Empower yourself with the knowledge to make informed food choices and take proactive steps toward managing stress for a healthier and more balanced life.

CHAPTER 12: MINDFUL EATING AND EMOTIONAL WELLNESS

Understanding Emotional Eating

Emotional eating is a common phenomenon that many individuals experience at some point in their lives. It involves using food to cope with or soothe emotional discomfort rather than eating for physical nourishment. In this chapter, we will delve into eating, its causes, and its impact on our physical and emotional well-being. By understanding emotional eating more deeply, we can develop strategies to manage it effectively and foster a healthier relationship with food.

Defining Emotional Eating:

Emotional vs. Physical Hunger: Differentiate between emotional and physical hunger to recognize the signs and cues of emotional eating.

Triggers and Emotional States: Explore common triggers for emotional eating, such as stress, boredom, loneliness, and sadness, and how specific emotions can lead to food cravings.

The Cycle of Emotional Eating:

Emotional Triggers: Understand the emotional triggers that initiate the cycle of emotional eating and how they can create a pattern of using food for comfort or distraction.

Temporary Relief vs. Long-Term Consequences: Recognize the temporary relief that emotional eating provides and the potential negative impact on overall health, weight management, and emotional well-being.

Addressing Emotional Eating:

Self-Awareness and Mindfulness: Learn techniques to cultivate self-awareness and mindfulness around eating habits, emotions, and triggers.

Emotional Regulation Strategies: Explore alternative strategies for coping with emotions, such as practicing relaxation techniques, engaging in physical activity, journaling, or seeking support from friends, family, or professionals.

Creating Healthy Coping Mechanisms: Develop a toolbox of healthy coping mechanisms to replace emotional eating, such as engaging in hobbies, practicing self-care, or seeking emotional support.

Nourishing Your Emotional Well-being:

Nutrient-Dense Foods for Mood Support: Discover foods rich in nutrients that support emotional well-being, including omega-3 fatty acids, magnesium, B vitamins, and antioxidants.

Balanced and Mindful Eating: Learn about the importance of balanced meals, adequate hydration, and mindful eating practices to support emotional stability and reduce the likelihood of emotional eating.

Cultivating a Healthy Relationship with Food:

Food as Nourishment: Shift the focus from using food solely for emotional comfort to viewing it as nourishment for the body and mind.

Developing a Positive Food Environment: Create an environment that supports healthy eating habits, including mindful grocery shopping, meal planning, and creating a peaceful dining environment.

Understanding emotional eating is crucial to developing a healthier relationship with food and managing emotional well-being effectively. By identifying emotional triggers, practicing self-awareness, and cultivating alternative coping mechanisms, we can break the cycle of emotional eating. Nourishing our bodies with nutrient-dense foods and adopting mindful eating practices support emotional stability and overall well-being. Remember, food should be enjoyed for nourishment and pleasure, not solely to cope with emotions. Take control of your emotional eating patterns and foster a healthier, balanced approach to food.

Mindful Eating Practices

In our fast-paced world, it's easy to fall into the trap of mindless eating, consuming meals and snacks without being present or aware of our food choices and eating patterns. Mindful eating offers a powerful antidote to this by inviting us to reconnect with the eating experience, fostering a deeper appreciation for food, and promoting a healthier relationship with nourishment. In this chapter, we will explore the concept of mindful eating and introduce practical strategies to incorporate it into your daily life.

What is Mindful Eating?

The Basics of Mindful Eating: Understand the core principles of mindful eating, including awareness, non-judgment, and presence.

Breaking the Cycle of Mindless Eating: Recognize the impact of mindless eating on our overall health and well-being and why cultivating mindful eating habits is beneficial.

The Mindful Eating Process:

Engaging the Senses: Explore how engaging your senses—sight, smell, taste, and texture—can enhance the eating experience and increase satisfaction.

Slowing Down: Learn the importance of slowing down during meals, savouring each bite, and allowing time for recognizing digestion and satiety cues.

Listening to Hunger and Fullness Cues: Develop an awareness of your body's hunger and fullness signals and learn to honour them without judgment.

Cultivating Mindful Eating Habits:

Meal Planning and Preparation: Discover how meal planning and preparation can support mindful eating by promoting intentionality and creating a positive food environment.

Mindful Grocery Shopping: Learn strategies for conscious grocery shopping, including making thoughtful food choices and being aware of the foods that nourish your body.

Eating with Awareness: Explore techniques to enhance your eating experience, such as practicing gratitude, chewing slowly, and removing distractions like electronic devices.

Emotional Awareness and Mindful Eating:

Recognizing Emotional Triggers: Understand how emotions influence our eating habits and differentiate between emotional and physical hunger.

Emotional Regulation: Develop strategies to navigate emotional eating triggers mindfully, such as engaging in alternative stress-relieving activities or seeking support.

Mindful Eating for Optimal Health:

Nourishing your Body: Discover the importance of choosing nutrient-dense foods that support your overall health and well-being.

Enjoyment and Pleasure: Embrace the joy of eating and savouring the flavours and textures of your meals.

Mindful eating is an invitation to slow down, tune in, and genuinely appreciate the nourishment our food provides. By cultivating mindful eating practices, we can develop healthier and more balanced relationships with food, enhance digestion and nutrient absorption, and foster a sense of satisfaction and well-being. Incorporate the principles of mindful eating into your daily life, and rediscover the joy and nourishment that comes from genuinely savouring each bite.

Promoting Emotional Wellness through Nutrition

Our emotional well-being is deeply intertwined with physical health; nutrition is crucial in supporting both. The foods we consume can impact our mood, energy levels, and overall mental well-being. This chapter will explore the connection between nutrition and emotional wellness and discuss how mindful food choices promote emotional balance and resilience.

The Gut-Brain Axis:

Understanding the Gut-Brain Connection: Explore the intricate relationship between the gut and the brain and how the gut microbiota influences our mood and emotional health.

The Role of Serotonin: Learn about serotonin, the "feel-good" neurotransmitter, and how its production is influenced by nutrition.

Nutrients for Emotional Well-being:

Omega-3 Fatty Acids: Discover the importance of omega-3 fatty acids for brain health and emotional well-being, and identify dietary sources.

B Vitamins: Understand the role of B vitamins in supporting cognitive function and managing stress, and learn which foods are rich in these nutrients.

Antioxidants: Explore the impact of oxidative stress on mental health and the role of antioxidants in reducing inflammation and promoting brain health.

Mood-Boosting Foods:

Whole Grains: Learn about the benefits of complex carbohydrates in promoting the production of serotonin and stabilizing blood sugar levels.

Leafy Greens and Cruciferous Vegetables: Discover the nutritional properties of these vegetables and their potential to support brain health and mood regulation.

Probiotic-Rich Foods: Explore the connection between gut health and emotional well-being, and identify fermented foods that nourish gut microbiota.

Balancing Blood Sugar Levels:

The Impact of Blood Sugar Imbalance: Understand how blood sugar fluctuations can contribute to mood swings, fatigue, and irritability.

Strategies for Balanced Blood Sugar: Learn practical tips for stabilizing blood sugar levels through balanced meals, portion control, and mindful eating.

Mindful Eating for Emotional Wellness:

Cultivating Awareness: Develop mindfulness around your eating habits, pay attention to hunger and fullness cues, and honour your body's needs.

Nourishing Self-Care: Explore the concept of self-care and how it relates to emotional wellness, and discover nourishing practices beyond food that support overall well-being.

By understanding the connection between nutrition and emotional wellness, we can make informed food choices that support our mental health and enhance our emotional resilience. Incorporating mood-boosting nutrients, balancing blood sugar levels, and practicing mindful eating can all contribute to greater emotional well-being. Embrace the power of nutrition as a tool for promoting emotional wellness and embark on a journey towards a healthier, happier, and more balanced life.

Recipes

Recipe 1: Rainbow Buddha Bowl

Ingredients:

- 1 cup cooked quinoa

- 1 cup roasted sweet potatoes, cubed

- 1 cup steamed broccoli florets

- 1 cup shredded carrots

- 1 cup sliced bell peppers (assorted colours)

- 1/2 cup sliced avocado

- 1/4 cup chickpeas (canned or cooked)

- 2 tablespoons tahini dressing

- Fresh cilantro for garnish

Instructions:

1. Arrange the cooked quinoa as the base of the bowl.

2. Arrange the roasted sweet potatoes, steamed broccoli, shredded carrots, sliced bell peppers, avocado, and chickpeas on top of the quinoa.

3. Drizzle the tahini dressing over the bowl.

4. Garnish with fresh cilantro.

5. Toss the ingredients together before enjoying this vibrant and nutritious Buddha bowl.

Recipe 2: Green Smoothie

Ingredients:

- 1 ripe banana

- 1 cup fresh spinach leaves

- 1/2 cup frozen mango chunks

- 1/2 cup almond milk (or any plant-based milk)

- 1 tablespoon chia seeds

- 1 tablespoon almond butter

- 1 teaspoon honey (optional, for sweetness)

Instructions:

1. Place all the ingredients in a blender.

2. Blend until smooth and creamy.

3. Adjust the consistency by adding more almond milk if desired.

4. Pour into a glass and enjoy this refreshing and nutrient-packed green smoothie.

Recipe 3: Quinoa Stuffed Bell Peppers

Ingredients:

- 4 bell peppers (assorted colors), tops cut off and seeds removed

- 1 cup cooked quinoa

- 1 cup black beans (canned or cooked)

- 1/2 cup corn kernels

- 1/2 cup diced tomatoes

- 1/2 cup diced red onion

- 1/2 cup shredded cheese (vegan or regular)

- 1 tablespoon olive oil

- 1 teaspoon cumin

- 1/2 teaspoon paprika

- Salt and pepper to taste

Instructions:

1. Preheat the oven to 375°F (190°C).

2. In a large mixing bowl, combine cooked quinoa, black beans, corn kernels, diced tomatoes, red onion, olive oil, cumin, paprika, salt, and pepper. Mix well.

3. Stuff the bell peppers with the quinoa mixture and place them in a baking dish.

4. Sprinkle shredded cheese on top of each stuffed bell pepper.

5. Bake in the preheated oven for 25-30 minutes or until the peppers are tender and the cheese is melted and slightly golden.

6. Remove from the oven and let them cool for a few minutes before serving. Enjoy this wholesome and flavorful dish.

Recipe 4: Mango Avocado Salad

Ingredients:

- 2 cups mixed salad greens

- 1 ripe mango, peeled and cubed

- 1 ripe avocado, peeled and sliced

- 1/4 cup red onion, thinly sliced

- 2 tablespoons chopped fresh cilantro

- Juice of 1 lime

- 1 tablespoon extra-virgin olive oil

- Salt and pepper to taste

Instructions:

1. In a large salad bowl, combine the mixed salad greens, cubed mango, sliced avocado, red onion, and chopped cilantro.

2. In a small bowl, whisk together the lime juice, olive oil, salt, and pepper to make the dressing.

3. Drizzle the dressing over the salad and toss gently to coat all the ingredients.

4. Serve immediately as a refreshing and nutritious side salad or light meal.

Recipe 5: Chocolate Chia Pudding

Ingredients:

1/4 cup chia seeds

- 1 cup unsweetened almond milk (or any plant-based milk)

- 1 tablespoon unsweetened cocoa powder

- 1 tablespoon maple syrup or honey

- 1/2 teaspoon vanilla extract

- Fresh berries or sliced bananas, for topping

Instructions:

1. In a bowl, whisk together the chia seeds, almond milk, cocoa powder, maple syrup or honey, and vanilla extract until well combined.

2. Let the mixture sit for about 5 minutes, then whisk again to prevent clumping.

3. Cover the bowl and refrigerate for at least 2 hours or overnight, allowing the chia seeds to absorb the liquid and create a pudding-like consistency.

4. Stir the mixture before serving to ensure even texture.

5. Top with fresh berries or sliced bananas for added flavor and enjoy this decadent yet nutritious chocolate chia pudding.

Conclusion

Embracing Holistic Nutrition for a Vibrant Life

In a world filled with various diet trends and quick-fix solutions, embracing holistic nutrition offers a refreshing approach to achieving optimal health and vitality. Holistic nutrition recognizes that true well-being goes beyond what we eat—it encompasses our lifestyle, mindset, and overall approach to life. By nourishing our bodies, minds, and spirits with intention and balance, we can experience a vibrant and fulfilling life. We will explore the principles and practices of holistic nutrition and learn how to incorporate them into our daily lives.

Understanding Holistic Nutrition:

Holistic Health Philosophy: Gain insight into the holistic health philosophy and understand its focus on the interconnectedness of body, mind, and spirit.

Holistic Approach to Nutrition: Explore the principles of holistic nutrition, including the importance of whole foods, mindful eating, and individualized dietary choices.

Nourishing the Body:

Nutrient-Dense Foods: Learn about the power of nutrient-dense foods that provide essential vitamins, minerals, and antioxidants for optimal health.

Balancing Macronutrients: Understand the role of carbohydrates, proteins, and fats in providing energy, supporting growth, and maintaining overall well-being.

Supporting Digestive Health: Discover the importance of a healthy gut and explore strategies to support digestion and nutrient absorption.

Cultivating a Balanced Mindset:

Mindful Eating Practices: Develop a mindful approach to eating by engaging all your senses, paying attention to hunger and fullness cues, and savouring each bite.

Managing Stress: Explore techniques to manage stress, such as relaxation exercises, meditation, and cultivating self-care practices that nourish your mental well-being.

Emotional Wellness: Understand the connection between emotions and eating habits, and learn strategies to promote emotional well-being and a positive relationship with food.

Nurturing the Spirit:

Finding Joy in Eating: Embrace the pleasure of eating by savouring flavours, engaging in social connections, and appreciating the nourishment food provides.

Connecting with Nature: Explore the benefits of connecting with nature and incorporating fresh, seasonal, and locally sourced foods into your diet.

Practicing Mind-Body Activities: Engage in mind-body practices like yoga, tai chi, or meditation to enhance overall well-being and foster a deeper mind-body connection.

Embracing holistic nutrition is an invitation to prioritize your health, well-being, and vitality. By nourishing your body with wholesome foods, fostering a balanced mindset, and nurturing your spirit, you can experience a vibrant and fulfilling life. Remember that holistic nutrition is a journey, and it's about finding what works best for you as an individual. Embrace the principles and practices of holistic nutrition, and let them guide you towards vibrant health, increased energy, and a profound sense of well-being.

Thank You for Embarking on This Nourishing Journey

Dear Reader,

I express my deepest gratitude for joining me on this transformative journey toward embracing holistic nutrition. By exploring the pages of "Alchemy of Nourishment: Unleashing the Magic of Holistic Nutrition," you have taken a significant step towards nourishing your body, mind, and spirit for a vibrant life.

Your dedication to seeking optimal health and wellness is commendable. Through this book, I have strived to provide valuable insights, practical guidance, and delicious recipes to empower you on your path to well-being. I hope the knowledge and inspiration within these pages will catalyze positive change in your life.

Remember, the magic of holistic nutrition lies not only in the foods we consume but also in the mindful choices we make, the connections we foster, and the love and compassion we cultivate for ourselves and others. This journey is not meant to be walked alone, and I am grateful to have you as a companion on this path.

As you navigate the chapters of this book, may you find empowerment, inspiration, and a deeper understanding of the intricate balance between nutrition and vitality. Let the alchemical nourishment processes guide you toward excellent health, radiance, and joy in all aspects of your life.

Thank you for investing your time, energy, and trust in "Alchemy of Nourishment." I wish that the wisdom you gain from these pages will nourish your body, ignite your spirit, and bring forth a profound transformation that lasts a lifetime.

With heartfelt gratitude,

Nancy Tran, RHN, CSCS

RESOURCES/ REFERENCES

Alcohol Consumption, Hypertension, and Cardiovascular Health Across the Life Course: There Is No Such Thing as a One-Size-Fits-All Approach.. https://www.repository.cam.ac.uk/handle/1810/283385

Infectious Diseases Acupuncture - Shenque Acupuncture. https://www.shenqueacupuncture.com/infectious-diseases-acupuncture/

Spirituality and Happiness | Mind to Body Yoga | 905-712-9642. https://mindtobody.ca/spirituality_happiness/

Episode 054 - Chrystal Evans Hurst, Author, The 28-Day Prayer Journey ·. https://thatmakestotalsense.com/podcast/episode-054-chrystal-evans-hurst-author-the-28-day-prayer-journey/

The Connection Between Food and Eye Health - Glenmore Landing Vision Center. https://www.glenmorevisioncenter.com/food-and-eye-health/

DarrenDaily Journal by DARREN HARDY –. https://store.darrenhardy.com/products/darrendaily-journal

Vegan Crush. https://maricelsvegancrush.com/food-education/

Talk One2One Student Assistance Program – Wellness at Cummings School. https://vetsites.tufts.edu/wellness/talk-one2one-student-assistance-program/

The Importance of a Balanced Diet for Women's Weight Loss - Youth Principles - Weight Loss Tips- Best weight loss tips. https://youthprinciples.com/the-importance-of-a-balanced-diet-for-womens-weight-loss/

Grocery Carts – Vitalcart. http://vitalcart.co/category/grocery-carts/

I'm trying to create a Referral for a Partner, but they're not showing up in the owner dropdown. What's going on? : Support Portal & Knowledge Base. https://help.channeltivity.com/support/solutions/articles/3000110827-i-m-trying-to-create-a-referral-for-a-partner-but-they-re-not-showing-up-in-the-owner-dropdown-what

Alps Natural Pureness Whole Earth Pork Dry Dog Food | tadaa!. https://tadaa.my/products/alpsnatural-dog-pork

https://www.bikehacks.com/things-cyclists-should-do/

Why bother with nutrition? - strivehealth.expert. https://www.strivehealth.expert/why-bother-with-nutrition/

The Shocking Truth About Pet Food: What You Need to Know. https://dontgetserious.com/the-shocking-truth-about-pet-food-what-you-need-to-know/

Community Data and Reports | Pueblo County. https://county.pueblo.org/public-health/community-data-and-reports

The Gut Microbiome and Mental Health: What You Need to Know → Healthy Weight Loss App | Lasta.app. https://lasta.app/the-gut-microbiome-and-mental-health-what-you-need-to-know/

Everything you need to know about Feel Moodtropics | Feel - Wellness, Reimagined. https://wearefeel.com/blogs/nutrition/everything-you-need-to-know-about-feel-moodtropics

5V Media | Blog - Our top tips to beat Blue Monday. https://www.weare5vmedia.com/media/our-top-tips-to-beat-blue-monday

Covid-19: Communicate your Reopening Plans to Customers Effectively. https://edifian.digital/covid-19-communicate-your-reopening-plans-to-customers-effectively/

Eat – hChoices. https://hchoices.com/healthier-happier-u/eat/

What are Macros and How Do I Count Them - Full Fitness. https://fullfitness.net/what-are-macros-and-how-do-i-count-them/

Environmental Allergy Symptoms. https://www.cchwyo.org/news/2020/june/environmental-allergy-symptoms/

When should you see a doctor for ADHD? - Drlogy. https://drlogy.com/question/when-should-you-see-a-doctor-for-adhd

Female Incontinence - Eramosa Physiotherapy. https://eramosaphysio.com/conditions/pelvic-floor-physiotherapy/female-incontinence/

Hot Yoga: An inside look – The Columbia Chronicle. https://columbiachronicle.com/4e080ec4-2c64-5de0-86d6-8fd63dff1c58

Do You Really Need Snow Tires? | AAA Club Alliance. https://cluballiance.aaa.com/the-extra-mile/articles/prepare/car/do-you-really-need-snow-tires

Benefits of Room Temperature Water Or Cold Water, Which One Is Better. https://www.epicwaterfilters.com/blogs/drip-quips/room-temperature-water-or-cold-water-which-one-is-better-for-you

Albumin Gene Targeting in Human Embryonic Stem Cells and Induced Pluripotent Stem Cells with Helper-Dependent Adenoviral Vector to Monitor Hepatic Differentiation - Institute of Molecular Embryology and Genetics, Kumamoto university. https://www.imeg.kumamoto-u.ac.jp/en/albumin-gene-targeting-in-human-embryonic-stem-cells-and-induced-pluripotent-stem-cells-with-helper-dependent-adenoviral-vector-to-monitor-hepatic-differentiation/

Kidney diagram with labels game quiz online. https://www.ecosystemforkids.com/games/kidney-diagram-with-labels.html

Foods High In Fiber: The Best Friends Of Weight-Loss Regimen. https://howtocure.com/foods-high-in-fiber/

Bermudagrass Suppression Methods for Oklahoma Home Gardens | Oklahoma State University. https://extension.okstate.edu/fact-sheets/bermudagrass-suppression-methods-for-oklahoma-home-gardens.html

Where can i get a cortisone shot for acne near me, oxandrolone dose | Profilo. https://www.studiomedicoecograficopavese.com/profile/nemets43/profile

Khadi Natural Herbal Handmade Pure Mint Soap - 125gm (Pack of 4) – Caresupp.in. https://caresupp.in/products/khadi-natural-herbal-handmade-pure-mint-soap-125gm-pack-of-4

Harmful Oral Health Effects of Beverages | Johnson Family Dentistry | Orlando Dentist. https://www.johnsonfamilydentistry.com/harmful-oral-health-effects-of-beverages/

Importance of Your Oral Health and Surprising ways to improve it - Smile Angels of Beverly Hills. https://smileangels.com/blog/dental-health/importance-of-your-oral-health-and-surprising-ways-to-improve-it/

My WellBeing Review 2023 - Matching Individuals With Therapists - Affiliates Maker. https://affiliatesmaker.com/my-wellbeing-review-2023/survey/

Finding A New You: Weight Loss Tips And Tricks. https://weightloss-review.biz/finding-a-new-you-weight-loss-tips-and-tricks-3/

What Do You Mean By Balanced Diet? » Gkbooks. https://gkbooks.in/web-stories/what-do-you-mean-by-balanced-diet/

Is Whole Foods Food Healthy? - ArthurHenrys. https://arthurhenrys.net/is-whole-foods-food-healthy/

Top 10 Best Meal Prep Services In Malaysia 2023 | Good-service. https://www.myweekendplan.asia/top-best-meal-prep-services-in-malaysia/

7 Foods That Are Proven to Increase Blood Flow. https://www.mayorboss.com/7-foods-that-are-proven-to-increase-blood-flow/

Tea and infusion with tropical fruits: our selection | Kusmi Tea. https://www.kusmitea.com/int/our-teas-and-herbal-teas/ingredient/tropical-fruits

Creamy cashew mayo — VEGANE VIBES. https://www.veganevibes.com/creamy-cashew-mayo/

Brain Health: How To Improve And Maintain | VINA-ACV – DRINK VINA. https://www.drinkvina.com/blogs/news/brain-health-improve-maintain

Black Sesame Seeds – VidiFood. https://vidifood.com/producto/black-sesame-seeds

Best Drink To Lower Blood Sugar. https://smasteri.com/stories/best-drink-to-lower-blood-sugar/

Holiday Baking with a Healthy Twist - ONIE Project. https://onieproject.org/holiday-baking-with-a-healthy-twist/

Healthy Dishes | Cleveland Tiffin. https://www.clevelandtiffin.com/about-1-1

The Best Superfoods for Women's Health. https://www.wildfoods.co/blogs/wild-blog/the-best-superfoods-for-womens-health

Police grapple with rise in cryptocurrency fraud - Financial news. https://financial-magazine.eu/2018/08/11/police-grapple-with-rise-in-cryptocurrency-fraud/

Can Cats Eat Dandelions? - HayFarmGuy. https://hayfarmguy.com/can-cats-eat-dandelions

Difference Between Guacamole and Avocado | Difference Between. http://www.differencebetween.net/object/comparisons-of-food-items/difference-between-guacamole-and-avocado/

"10 Superfoods You Should Be Eating for Optimal Health" – Toadstoollabs. https://toadstoollabs.com/blogs/news/10-superfoods-you-should-be-eating-for-optimal-health

Vegan Chia Seed Pancakes - YouEatPlants.com. https://youeatplants.com/vegan-chia-seed-pancakes/

15 Chocolate Recipes That Are Good For You – Creative Healthy Family. https://www.creativehealthyfamily.com/15-chocolate-recipes-that-are-actually-good-for-you/

Couscous vs Quinoa | Organic Facts. https://www.organicfacts.net/couscous-vs-quinoa.html

Top 10 Most Useful Herbs. https://www.vibhealthy.com/2023/01/top-10-most-useful-herbs.html

Cod and Asparagus - wellnesssleuth. https://wellnesssleuth.com/cod-and-asparagus/

herbal - Women Want Wellness. https://www.womenwantwellness.org/tag/herbal/

Learn the health benefits of cold brew coffee – GoodBrew. https://goodbrew.ie/blogs/news/health-benefits-of-drinking-coffee

Nutrition | Rensselaer County, NY. https://www.rensco.com/295/Nutrition

Five Superfood Tips. – KUMA Knives. https://kumaknives.com/blogs/blog/five-superfood-tips

Open Source Sustainable House Designs That Anyone Can Build – InApps Technology 2022 - InApps. https://www.inapps.net/open-source-sustainable-house-designs-that-anyone-can-build-inapps-technology-2022/

Can you trust the labels on your herbal supplements? | Bickerton Law Group, LLLP. https://www.bsdsblog.com/2017/08/can-you-trust-the-labels-on-your-herbal-supplements/

Part 1: Happiness; Chapter 5:Transforming Suffering into Joy [5.1] | Soka Gakkai (global). https://www.sokaglobal.org/resources/study-materials/buddhist-study/the-wisdom-for-creating-happiness-and-peace/chapter-5-1.html

What Exactly are Carbohydrates? | 8fit. https://8fit.com/nutrition/what-are-carbohydrates/

Keto flu - QI-Keto. https://qi-keto.com/road-to-keto/keto-flu/

Role of Fruits and Vegetables in Healthy Living and Longevity. https://www.blog.joyscore.co/role-of-fruits-and-vegetables-in-healthy-living-and-longevity/

Why do plants need phosphorus? [Top 5 Reasons]. https://gardenerideas.com/why-do-plants-need-phosphorus/

Burdock Root 2 – Sacred Oak Apothecary. https://sacredoakapothecary.com/blogs/herbs/burdock-root-2

4 Weight Loss Supplements You Need. https://uk.kaged.com/blogs/supplementation/5-weight-loss-supplements-you-need

Benefits Of Superfoods | Most 6 Popular Superfoods. https://apnewscorner.com/superfoods/

Leadership in Veterinary Medicine | Veterian Key. https://veteriankey.com/tag/leadership-in-veterinary-medicine/

immune system | Nancy Guberti, M.S., C.N.. https://nancyguberti.com/tag/immune-system/

10 Foods Help Reduce Joint And Back Pain - Blog - HealthifyMe. https://www.healthifyme.com/blog/web-stories/foods-help-joint-and-back-pain/

Biofortification: A weapon against hidden hunger. | Abstract. https://www.biomedres.info/abstract/biofortification-a-weapon-against-hidden-hunger-21450.html

Centrum Silver Adults 50+ 125 TABS. https://www.coffeedrinksnmore.com/en/home/42-centrum-silver-adults-50-125-tabs.html

Interaction of drugs with Vitamin D, Magnesium, Vitamin B12, Selenium, etc – Dec 2018 | VitaminDWiki. https://vitamindwiki.com/tiki-index.php?page=Interaction+of+drugs+with+Vitamin+D%2C+Magnesium%2C+Vita

Vitamins | Biesterfeld AG. https://www.biesterfeld.com/en/de/product/vitamins/

Leadership in Veterinary Medicine | Veterian Key. https://veteriankey.com/tag/leadership-in-veterinary-medicine/

Brewer's yeast - immunostimulator and antioxidant. https://arolife.bg/en/produkt/brewers-yeast/

The 3 Best B Vitamin Complex (#1 will WOW you!). https://www.wowzzzersreviews.com/best-b-vitamin-complex/

Guide to the Coumadin Diet: A Comprehensive Guide for Dieters. https://www.geekloveshealth.com/guide-to-the-coumadin-diet/

Best Whole House Water Filter to Remove Fluoride and Chlorine Reviews. https://homeintakes.com/best-whole-house-water-filter/

What Are Adaptogens? – Instil Natural Living. https://instilbeing.com/pages/what-are-adaptogens

5 Surprising Ways Your Diet Affects Your Gut Health - Armygymnastics | Health | Fitness. https://armygymnastics.com/5-surprising-ways-your-diet-affects-your-gut-health/

Wellbeing - My Fermented Foods. https://myfermentedfoods.com/category/wellbeing/

Food loss and waste in a changing environment — Research@WUR. https://research.wur.nl/en/publications/food-loss-and-waste-in-a-changing-environment

The Two Healing Ingredients In Every OWL Broth Recipe – OWL Venice. https://www.owlvenice.com/blogs/news/our-secret-healing-ingredients-in-every-owl-broth-recipe

What About Leaky Gut Syndrome | Universal Health Products. https://universal-health-products.com/what-about-leaky-gut-syndrome/embed/

3 Secrets To Thriving Thyroid Health From A Nutritional Therapist! | NutriRise. https://nutririse.com/blogs/health-nutrition-3/3-secrets-to-thriving-thyroid-health-from-a-nutritional-therapist

Leadership in Veterinary Medicine | Veterian Key. https://veteriankey.com/tag/leadership-in-veterinary-medicine/

Coverting Stem Cells into Insulin Producing Islets | ISCRM. https://iscrm.uw.edu/stories/promoting-cell-growth-in-the-pancreas/

Fasted Cardio May Be the Key to Burning Fat! - LAVYON. https://lavyon.com/en/fasted-cardio-may-be-the-key-to-burning-fat/

Eating around the holidays - a guide for cyclists | Team EF Coaching. https://www.teamefcoaching.com/blog/eating-around-the-holidays/

Exercise – Park Run. https://parkrun.ae/category/exercise/

Top 10 Foods For Health For Your Diet Health Beauty And Fitness. https://diet65.com/web-stories/health-tips-top-10-foods-for-health/

12-Bar Variety Pack | Real Food Bars, Vegan Protein Bars. https://realfoodbar.com/product/variety-pack

Xylitol – Frē Man. https://www.fremanusa.com/pages/xylitol-extract

This Popular Breakfast Food May Be Increasing Your Cancer Risk, New Study Suggests — Eat This Not That. https://www.eatthis.com/news-eggs-may-increase-cancer-risk-study/

Informational | CORE PT & Pilates. https://coreptpilates.com/category/educational/informational/

The Dangers of Anabolic Steroid Use for Women - manvsweight. https://manvsweight.com/the-dangers-of-anabolic-steroid-use-for-women/

Robert Whytt - Wikipedia. https://en.wikipedia.org/wiki/Robert_Whytt

xtra herbal. https://www.xtraherbal.com/product/277033/Yogi-Tea,-Relaxed-Mind,-Caffeine-Free,-16-Tea-Bags,-1.27-oz-%2836-g%29

Enjoying Your Weight Loss Success And The New Freedoms You Have | SlimFast. https://slimfast.com/health-beauty/enjoying-your-newfound-freedom/

Meditation for Weight Loss Program: Lose Weight Fast | Meditation App. https://mindtastik.com/meditation-for-weight-loss-program-lose-weight-fast/

Women's Bodies, Women's Wisdom By: Dr. Christiane Northrup. https://kellymcnelis.com/womens-bodies-womens-wisdom-by-dr-christiane-northrup/

Solitary Fears: the Fear of Being Alone - Phobious. https://phobious.com/solitary-fears-the-fear-of-being-alone/

Higher Order Functions | springerprofessional.de. https://www.springerprofessional.de/en/higher-order-functions/17050752

Cheryl Gunraj - Evexía by Design. https://www.evexiabydesign.com/me/cheryl-gunraj/

This Popular Breakfast Food May Be Increasing Your Cancer Risk, New Study Suggests — Eat This Not That. https://www.eatthis.com/news-eggs-may-increase-cancer-risk-study/

Unshakable Faith - Faiths Corresponding Action - Highway Community Church. https://highwaycommunity.com/unshakable-faith-faiths-corresponding-action/

Heart-Healthy Recipes for Diabetes. https://www.diabetesfoodhub.org/articles/heart-healthy-recipes-for-diabetes.html

Diet Changes To Make If You Have Stomach Problems. https://www.elitedaily.com/wellness/diet-changes-stomach-problems/1682315

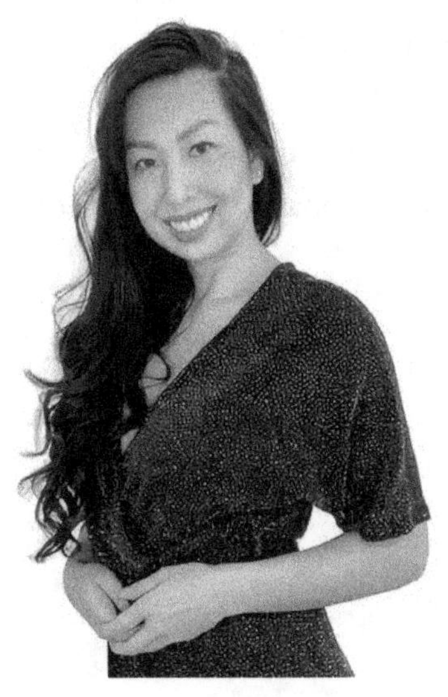

About the Author

Nancy is a certified strength and conditioning specialist and registered holistic nutritionist dedicated to helping individuals achieve their health and wellness goals. With a background in accounting and finance, she experienced struggles with weight, fatigue, and overall health, which sparked her passion for nutrition.

After graduating from the Canadian School of Natural Nutrition, Nancy combines her fitness and holistic nutrition expertise to empower others on their wellness journeys. As a natural health advisor and store manager at Nature's Signature, she provides personalized guidance on supplements and wellness products.

With a solid commitment to practicing what she preaches, Nancy embraces a healthy lifestyle while balancing it with other aspects of life. Her clients appreciate her accountability, reliability, and unwavering support as she helps them break bad habits and improve their well-being.

Nancy is thrilled to share her knowledge and experiences with readers, offering practical advice and inspiration to embrace holistic nutrition for a vibrant life. She hopes to empower individuals to take charge of their health and discover the transformative power of nourishing their bodies and minds through her writing.

Read more at holisticpharmacyandnutrition.com.

www.ingramcontent.com/pod-product-compliance
Lightning Source LLC
Chambersburg PA
CBHW061539120726
48001CB00004B/1637